Educating Yourself About Alcohol and Drugs

A PEOPLE'S PRIMER

Revised Edition

Educating Yourself About Alcohol and Drugs

A PEOPLE'S PRIMER

Revised Edition

Marc Alan Schuckit, M.D.

Illustrations by
Dena Leigh Schuckit

Plenum Trade • New York and London

Library of Congress Cataloging-in-Publication Data

Schuckit, Marc Alan, 1944-
    Educating yourself about alcohol and drugs : a people's primer /
Marc Alan Schuckit ; illustrations by Dena Leigh Schuckit. -- Rev.
ed.
        p.   cm.
    Includes bibliographical references and index.
    ISBN 0-306-45783-0
    1. Drug abuse. 2. Alcoholism. 3. Narcotic addicts-
-Rehabilitation. 4. Alcoholics--Rehabilitation.
HV5801.S363 1998
613.8--dc21   97-43209
                                                                   CIP

Cover Illustration by Dena Leigh Schuckit

ISBN 0-306-45783-0

© 1998, 1995 Marc A. Schuckit
Plenum Press is a Division of Plenum Publishing Corporation
233 Spring Street, New York, N.Y. 10013-1578
http://www.plenum.com

10 9 8 7 6 5 4 3 2 1

Printed in the United States of America

Neither this book, nor anything else that I've managed to accomplish, would have been possible without the love, support, and wonderful common sense of my lifetime partner and best friend, Judy. Through her I have learned my most important lessons in life, and her love is the source of my inspiration and strength.

Preface to the Entire Text

Some General Thoughts

This book was written to help people. My goal is to give the best possible information about drug and alcohol problems in the most straightforward manner possible. I hope this text will be used by people who are trying to decide whether or not they, or a loved one, have a problem with alcohol or drugs and to consider what might be done about it.

The thoughts offered here grew out of my work as both a researcher and the director of two alcohol and drug treatment programs. For thirty years I have worked with patients, friends, and colleagues who face possible drug problems. The questions asked by these important people in my life and by those around them made me realize there was no standard book based on solid data (not just opinions) for them to turn to. This problem is even more troubling in recent years because, as financial support for those problems has become scarce, it has become more and more difficult to enter treatment. I hope to fill some of that void.

I believe that, given enough information, people generally make rational decisions. When a person is trying to assess whether a drug or alcohol problem exists, and what to do to get help if one does, the best road to take might not always be obvious at first reading or thinking. However, with time the thoughts percolate and eventually a plan of action is likely to appear.

The Book Has Two Major Parts

To me, the two key ingredients for a successful recovery are, first, understanding as much as possible about one's situation, and, second, identifying the choice of actions one can take to move toward recovery. Therefore, this text is divided into two parts. The first offers information about what substances are, some thought about what they do to you, and a discussion of some of the risks you face when you take them. Part II offers detailed information about how steps to recovery can begin, what is likely to happen during treatment, and the importance of continuing care after the initial more intense efforts have occurred.

Several Types of Readers

The fact that you have picked up this book and are skimming the preface means that you have some potential need. Some of you are concerned about your own alcohol or drug use and need to make some important decisions. For others, someone you care about is having severe problems and you want to help. For yet others, nothing personal is involved, and you are "studying" to advance your career or because this is an interesting and potentially important topic for society in general.

I attempt to meet these different needs in two major ways. The first is to offer useful information that is a melding of data and clinical experience, giving the information in a straightforward way that is as free of jargon and technical words as I can get. The second major goal is to offer information that is as practical as possible, beginning each chapter with a brief statement of what it is trying to accomplish and ending with a brief summary about what was said. What lies between is the information offered in more detail, often with a presentation of both pros and cons.

Those readers who desire more detail can turn to the reference lists at the end of some chapters and the suggested readings. There is also a data-driven companion medical text that I have written that parallels much of the information offered here, *Drug and Alcohol Abuse: A Clinical Guide to Diagnosis and Treatment*, 4th Edition (New York, Plenum Medical Book Company, 1995).

Emotional texture, in addition to the words, is offered through original illustrations that were developed specifically for this book. Sometimes, spending a bit of time reflecting over these prints can bring home points that the words alone can't adequately describe.

Finally, the version of this book in your hand has been modified from the original published in 1995. Our goal has been to decrease the cost by printing with a soft cover and by deleting the original section on expanded readings from an appendix. While we were at it, we updated some of the additional readings at the end of the chapters and changed the front cover. However, the basic information and goals remain the same.

I owe a debt of gratitude to my editor, Mariclaire Cloutier, for her advice and friendship, without which this version would have never seen the light of day.

I hope that by this point you have decided that the text has something to offer you. This is as good a time as any to begin the process.

Contents

Preface to Part I

What are drugs of abuse, what do they do to you, and what prices do you pay for using them? It seems to me that the answers to these questions are essential if you want to make decisions about whether a substance problem exists and what might be done about it.

Chapter 1 attempts to teach you about what drugs are and explores the related concepts, such as tolerance and dependence, that you need to understand. Chapter 2 moves beyond these general statements to a more specific listing of the 250 or so substances people might use for a "high." By placing the substances into seven or so categories, you will learn how members within each category share many properties, including how they make you feel. The third and final chapter of Part I builds upon this information to give an overview of the wide range of prices you pay for substance use.

This is really the more straightforward section of the book. Much of what I offer here is the result of solid, dependable research. It is only after understanding the basic information regarding the characteristics of drugs and how they make you feel that you can make decisions about any problems you or anyone around you might have.

1

Chemicals Help Make Us What We Are

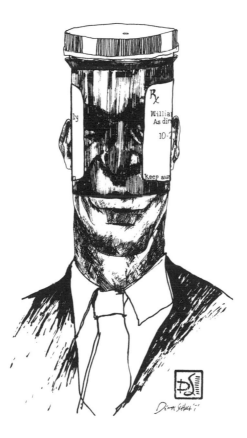

Figure 1.1. Throughout this text I do all I can to deal with the complex nature of much of the information being offered. Some of the lessons that need to be learned have an important emotional component. This creates a situation where words alone are not enough. As a result, most chapters have an illustration in the form of an original illustration developed specifically for the book. The goal is to try to present a representation of some of the emotional content of the basic message as a complement to the text offerings. Chapter 1 is the first step in your exploration of whether alcohol or drugs might be causing you problems or might be a danger for someone close to you. In order to understand the dangers of most substances of abuse, it is important first to understand their impact on the way your brain functions. One essential element of normal brain activity is the chemical makeup of brain tissue and the way that the chemicals of the brain (neurochemicals) carry out the work of communication from one cell to another. This illustration demonstrates how important chemicals are to normal brain functioning and the impact that alcohol and other drugs can have on this essential body system.

Goals

Notice that it is the chemicals inside your brain that help make you feel and act the way you do. All of the substances of abuse (that term is used to include both alcohol and all other drugs used deliberately to cause a "high") are chemicals that get into your body, find their way to your brain, and, as the result of a variety of different mechanisms, change how you feel. These drugs almost always interact, and interfere, with normal body chemicals. So, in order to understand what drugs of abuse do to you and to your chemical makeup, you must know something about how the brain works.

When you stop to think about it, the functioning of your entire body involves one series of chemical reactions after the other. Just as biochemical reactions govern how your liver and kidneys function, chemical reactions have also been identified as the essential mode of operation of your brain and the rest of your nervous system, including your spinal column and the nerves to your hands and feet. Therefore, it makes good sense that a substance taken to change how you feel must do so, at least in part, by altering the chemical reactions that go on inside of your head on a moment-to-moment basis. In fact, the actions of these substances might be similar in many ways to some of the longer-lasting chemical alterations that appear to contribute to forms of mental illness, such as major depression or schizophrenia.

The overall goal of this chapter is to put substances of abuse into some perspective. Although these drugs (including alcohol) differ in many important ways, they do share some basic properties. Understanding more about both the similarities and differences among drugs helps you to realize what is going on in your brain as a result of drug taking.

Before going into the specifics of each type of drug discussed in Chapter 2, you need to review how drugs act. The sections of this chapter review properties common to almost all substances of abuse. This information includes a definition of drugs, how they get to the brain, and some general aspects of how they change brain functioning. It discusses how these drugs alter how you feel and the concepts of psychological and physical dependence.

What Drugs Are and How They Are Taken

What Drugs Are

We all know what a drug is—it is just a bit difficult to put the concept into words. These are substances (that is, chemicals) that enter your body, find their way into your bloodstream, and are transported to the brain. In order to be substances that you desire, they change how you feel, often causing a floating sensation, either an intensification or a dulling of your perception of your senses, usually altering your level of alertness (either up or down), and sometimes decreasing physical pain. The final result is some "desired effect" that in one way or another gives a level of pleasure, or at least relief from discomfort. If you value these experiences, you are likely to use the drug again, and might even seek out the substance in spite of the prices you have to pay in money, time, discomfort, social or work impairment, or the potential of long-term damage to the body.

How Substances Find Their Way to the Brain

All substances of abuse have major actions in the brain. The methods by which they find their way into the body and then into the bloodstream in order to be transported to the brain are quite diverse and can impact on how rapidly and how intensely their actions are felt. At the same time, each type of administration involves some unique dangers.

Drugs that Can Be Inhaled

Taking some substances is as easy as breathing. The solvents or inhalants (like gasoline, toluene, and paint thinner) and gases like freon, nitrous oxide (laughing gas), and amyl and butyl nitrite ("poppers") are all taken in by inhaling. Once in the lungs, the substances rapidly dissolve in the rich blood supply. Then only a matter of seconds is required to go from the lungs to the heart and on to the brain. Therefore, it is not surprising that when a drug is easily inhaled, it is likely to cause a very quick and intense intoxication.

Some other substances are not naturally found in a gas-like state but are easily converted to this rapid-acting form. These include the nicotine in tobacco smoke, the active ingredient in any of the forms of cannabinols (including marijuana, hashish, and ganja), and the various "smokable" forms of opium and cocaine. Regarding the latter, the major reason for developing freebase cocaine and the "rock" or "crack" forms of this drug (the latter are names that only relate to the west or east coast of the United States—not different drugs) is to allow for efficient melting at relatively low temperatures so that the drug can be inhaled after burning in a pipe.

Opium, the direct product of the opium poppy plant and the base drug from which heroin and morphine are synthesized, can also be taken by smoking. This was the usual method of getting an opiate into the body in the infamous "opium dens" of China in the 19th century. However, because directly smoking heroin (as opposed to opium) in a pipe is an inefficient method of administration (most of the heroin is not burned up in the smoke), it wasn't until relatively recent years that an alternate form of inhaling burnt heroin became popular. This approach is called "chasing the dragon." Here, heroin is carefully heated on aluminum foil, and the wisps of white smoke (that look a bit like a dragon) are chased or inhaled through a straw or pipe. This form of administration is of increasing popularity in other parts of the world, especially Britain, and many American opiate addicts have recently learned of it. It is a more efficient mechanism of producing a high than eating heroin directly and avoids all of the dangers of IV use (such as AIDS, hepatitis, and endocarditis). Of course, this does nothing to avoid the other severe dangers associated with opiates, such as the possibility of death by overdose and the probability of physical addiction. Inhaling drugs has its own set of *problems*. One difficulty involves the local action that the substance can have in the lungs, producing irritation that can lead first to a cough and then to chronic bronchitis. In addition, some of these substances (for example, tobacco and marijuana smoke) are loaded with both cancer-causing agents and other chemicals that can destroy the structure of the lungs and produce emphysema, resulting in deadly long-term problems.

Drugs Taken by Needle

Some substances can be easily absorbed when inserted by a needle under the skin (subcutaneously or subQ). This produces a rate of transmission into the bloodstream that is slower than smoking, but usually faster than swallowing. The procedure, sometimes called "skin popping," is especially likely to be used for some forms of opiates, such as heroin.

For most people, however, using a needle is a way of getting the drug directly into the bloodstream. This intravenous or IV route involves injecting the substance directly into a vein, where (in a matter of minutes) it flows to the heart, lungs, and then to the brain. Because so much drug can be injected so quickly, this results in a very fast onset of an intense intoxication. In order to be taken this way, the substance must be easily dissolved in a liquid. Intravenous drugs include several types of opiates (including heroin and Demerol or meperidine), some forms of cocaine, some brain depressants (including barbiturates and some benzodiazepines like Valium or diazepam), and some forms of amphetamines (especially methamphetamine or "speed").

The *dangers* involved with IV drug administration are frightening. Even if totally clean needles are used, the impact on the brain of such large doses of drugs so quickly can cause severe illness and even death. For example, amphetamines and cocaine in high enough doses cause brain blood vessels to clamp down or go into spasm, which can precipitate a stroke in someone who is already having some level of problems with his or her blood vessels. High doses of any of the substances can cause vital brain centers either to become overstimulated or to shut down, with a resulting rapid death. When amphetamines and cocaine are involved, the overstimulation results in a very high blood pressure (which further increases the chances of a stroke), a very high body temperature, a rapid and unstable heartbeat pattern that can cause a heart attack, and the possibility of potentially fatal convulsions. Heavy loads of opiates and brain depressants are likely to shut down the breathing center, the part of the brain that regulates the heartbeat, and cause a rapid drop in blood pressure—any of which can, by themselves, cause death.

The stakes increase dramatically if nonsterile needles or syringes are used. In this case, in addition to the dangers of the specific drug, bacteria and viruses can rapidly find their way into the bloodstream in such huge amounts that they can produce severe and potentially fatal infections of the liver (hepatitis). For other people, the bacteria accumulate on the valves of the heart (a condition called bacterial endocarditis) and subsequently destroy the ability of the heart to regulate the in- and out-flow of blood, with potentially lethal consequences. Repeated exposure to needles shared with someone who has acquired immune deficiency syndrome (AIDS) almost inevitably leads to the disease itself, as demonstrated by the greater than 80% of IV drug users in some large metropolitan areas who have contracted the disorder. This latter case not only means a most difficult death for the needle user but also exposes sexual partners to the same fate.

Drugs Taken by Snorting (Insufflation)

A few drugs are so easily absorbed into the body that putting them in contact with any body area that has a lot of blood flow is likely to result in transmission through the blood to the brain. The lining of the nose, mouth, and throat are examples of body tissues rich in blood supply. Therefore, some drugs, notably forms of amphetamines, cocaine, and opiates, can be "snorted" in powder form into the nose (a procedure called **insufflation**) for fairly rapid absorption. The resulting high comes on a bit slower than with smoking or IV use, but it is more rapid than the high that occurs with swallowing substances.

The *problems* associated uniquely with snorting relate mostly to the effects that the drug has on the tissues it touches. Cocaine and amphetamine, in general, cause blood vessels to constrict, and the vessels in the lining of the nose are no exception. Therefore, many people who snort these drugs develop abscesses and local sores in the nose. Sometimes, blood supply can become so restricted that the death of tissue in the nose produces a hole in the septum separating the two nostrils.

Drugs Taken by Swallowing

As one would expect, this is the most common way of ingesting substances. Among the drugs of abuse most often taken orally are those originally marketed by pharmaceutical companies to be taken in pill form, including some of the stimulants (for example, diet pills and most forms of amphetamines), and almost all of the depressant-type drugs (barbiturates like Seconal, also called secobarbital, and the benzodiazepines, for example, Valium). Almost all of the opiates on the market are likely to be abused in pill form, including Demerol (meperidine), Methadone, Percodan (oxycodone), Talwin (pentazocine), and even Darvon (propoxyphene). Of course, other drugs can be easily absorbed from the digestive tract, including alcohol, the hallucinogens such as lysergic acid diethylamide (LSD), and even marijuana.

When taken orally, drugs go through the stomach and into the small intestine where there is usually a delay of anywhere from ten minutes to an hour before the drug is absorbed into the bloodstream. The blood flow from the intestine first passes through the liver (where some of the drug is destroyed) before coming back to the heart. Once there, it takes only minutes to pump the blood to the lungs, back to the heart, and up to the brain. Some substances, however, are either destroyed by the acids and other digestive juices in the stomach or are not well absorbed from the intestine. Thus, for example, most drug takers prefer not to swallow any of the forms of cocaine and most of the forms of heroin.

It is likely that the *dangers* uniquely associated with swallowing drugs are probably less than those seen with the other forms of drug administration. Some substances, such as alcohol, can cause irritation to the esophagus, or food tube, or to the stomach. Some cause potentially extensive damage to the liver, although this would be true no matter how they had been taken into the body, because all of the blood sooner or later is filtered through this organ.

Drugs Taken by Other Methods

As you might guess, the mechanisms used to get drugs into the body, and therefore to the brain, can be quite diverse. Therefore, some drugs are taken by rectum in a suppository-like form, some are absorbed from under the tongue (sublingual), and others—like some forms of LSD—can even be taken through the skin as a type of skin patch. However, most drugs of abuse are taken into the body through the four routes described above.

How Drugs Change the Brain

I could begin this section by telling you that the details of how these drugs work are too complicated to be easily explained. The truth of the matter is that the brain itself is so complex that drug actions are not completely understood.

This complexity is the result of the fact that most of the drugs produce different, and sometimes even opposite, effects in different areas of the brain, all at the same time. So, understanding how a specific drug changes a specific chemical under one unique set of circumstances might do little to help us understand which of the many changes seen in many different brain chemicals are *key* to producing intoxication or long-term consequences. To make matters even more complex, what the drug does to the brain the first time it is taken is different from what is likely to occur with repeated use. These effects, in turn, are frequently quite different (often the opposite) from what is likely to be observed as the brain attempts to readjust after drug taking is stopped.

It is, however, possible to discuss some generalities.

Some Drugs Affect the Nerve Cell Membrane

The cells of the body operate, at least in part, by selectively allowing certain substances such as sodium, chloride, and calcium to flow in and others to flow out of themselves. This process is regulated by the membrane (or "skin") surrounding the cell.

Obviously, anything that alters the policing of what comes and what goes can impact the state of cell functioning. Some drugs have at least some of their effects on the membrane of nerve cells or neurons.

The classical example is alcohol. The membranes or "skins" of nerve cells are loaded with fats in the form of cholesterol, and the condition of these fats is an essential part of the control of the flow of substances into and out of the cell. Alcohol is believed to change the level of rigidity of the cell membrane, at least in part by its actions on the fat. As the membrane becomes less rigid, the cell loses some of its protection from surrounding chemicals. This might impair the functioning of the cell and contribute to feelings of intoxication. The strength of this effect on the membrane and its course over time correlate in many ways with the intoxicating and other clinical effects of alcohol.

Some Drugs Change Structures Attached to the Cells (Receptors)

Brain cells do not really touch one another. Rather, there is a tiny space, called the **synapse,** between cells. Therefore, for one cell to affect another, it releases chemicals that rapidly flow across the empty space to impact on the second cell. These chemicals are received by tiny "feelers" (called **receptors**) that then become stimulated, causing the desired change in the second cell. Whether by luck or by design, some of the drugs of abuse have direct and very potent effects on specific receptors. An excellent example of this occurs with the opiates, including heroin. Perhaps as a means to control normal levels of pain, many brain cells have receptors that are specifically sensitive to naturally occurring opium-like substances in the body, substances called endorphins and enkephalins. These receptors not only are strongly affected by the body's natural opiates but are vulnerable to the effects of opiates such as heroin or prescription pain killers such as propoxyphene (Darvon). Once stimulated, the receptors set off a series of changes in the cell, altering the normal ability of the brain to perceive pain messages and decreasing feelings of physical pain. The dangers here occur not as a direct result of receptor stimulation but because of how the body changes to resist repeated stimulation by heroin (a process of tolerance discussed below). The result of tolerance is the need for higher doses of the drug to get the same effect. Therefore, at least in part because of these receptor changes, people can build up a need for very high doses of opiates, such high levels that the blood pressure can drop and breathing rates can slow down to dangerous levels. A related problem is that when the drug use is stopped, the changes in these receptors can produce symptoms of withdrawal, as discussed below.

A second example of brain receptor changes comes with one of the several brain effects of the benzodiazepines, including diazepam (Valium). A number of areas of the brain are rich in receptors sensitive to the effects of the group of drugs known as benzodiazepines, which include all of the Valium-type drugs. All of these share the ability to help people sleep, to rapidly decrease levels of anxiety, and to produce feelings of muscle relaxation. No one knows for sure which of the body's own chemicals affect these receptors, but it is agreed that many of the intoxicating effects of the benzodiazepines occur through drug-induced changes in the receptors in different areas of the brain. The dangers of tolerance and a subsequent withdrawal syndrome are similar to those described for opiates.

It is also likely that many other drug effects occur because of receptor changes. Good candidates for these mechanisms of effect are specific receptors that are sensitive to phencyclidine (PCP), and others that might also change with hallucinogens such as LSD. There are even hypothesized receptor changes in the presence of the marijuana-type drugs.

Some Drugs Operate by Directly Changing Brain Chemicals

There are probably hundreds of natural chemicals that are present in the brain and that can be released from one cell to travel across the space between cells (a synapse) to stimulate the next cell. Some of these substances (called neurotransmitters or neurochemicals) resemble adrenalin and result in increased brain activity, whereas others tend to decrease overall brain actions with resulting sedation and fatigue. For some drugs of abuse, the mechanisms of action are the direct result of their effects on these natural brain chemicals.

There are many examples of drugs of abuse that alter the levels of these chemical transmitters. Some, like cocaine and amphetamines, have major actions on the levels of adrenalin-like neurotransmitters, including norepinephrine and dopamine. Others, especially brain depressants such as alcohol and the Valium-type drugs, seem to have at least some of their major effects through changes they produce in more sedating-type brain chemicals, including gamma aminobutyric acid (abbreviated as GABA). Yet others have a huge impact on additional brain transmitters such as serotonin and acetylcholine.

A Mini Recap

For many, it is enough to know that a drug gets to the brain, changes how you feel, and can cause problems. For some others, however, it helps to take some of the mystery away from drugs by demonstrating that they all have effects on the brain by altering the chemicals that are already there. The final result is a brain that is trying to carry on normal day-to-day activities while the drugs are pushing buttons that make it difficult to keep things in balance. The consequences are likely to be mood swings, changes in judgment, and other signs that this critical body organ, the brain, is not functioning in an optimal way. The next section briefly reviews some processes common to almost all drugs of abuse, regardless of their specific mode of chemical operation.

Drugs Change How We Feel, with Predictable Results

Psychological Dependence or Addiction

Although drugs change how you feel, there are only a limited number of overall effects that you can expect. Among other things, a substance might make you happy or sad, relaxed or nervous, confused, or make you think that you are receiving stimulation in one of your senses (a hallucination). Any change is likely to be the result of some alteration in a part of the cell membrane, a receptor, or a brain chemical.

Almost by definition, if a substance is to become a problem, one must view these drug-induced changes as pleasurable, or at least desirable. If that were not the case (for example if the only action of drug were to make you go blind—even temporarily), most people would not be likely to continue using the drug. Without some level of reward, you certainly would not be likely to continue to put forth an effort to get the substance if it were causing problems in your life.

It is these overall pleasurable (or at least desirable) drug effects that cause a phenomenon known as **psychological addiction or dependence.** Notice that in almost every phase of this text I will be using the words addiction and dependence to mean basically the same thing. Here, psychological dependence indicates that after you have some experience with the substance, you find yourself wanting to take it again. This desire might be later the same night or maybe in two weeks, but the result is the same. The drug or alcohol has acquired some value to you, and you are willing to pay a price to continue the experience.

If the price you are willing to pay is relatively low or if the substance you are considering has few dangers, then psychological dependence would hardly be a cause for major concern. On the other hand, when you are willing to spend a significant amount of money to pay for the substance, exert a great deal of your time and effort in order to get the chemical, or are willing to experience problems in your job, get in trouble legally, and let your relationships with people you care about suffer because of drug use, you have developed psychological dependence.

Every substance mentioned in this text is capable, under certain conditions, of producing some level of psychological addiction. One of the difficulties is that the greater the level of psychological addiction, the greater the reluctance to admit either that you have problems or that the drug is associated with the difficulties. You can desire the substance so much that you are willing to deny, even to yourself, that you are paying a price, a process appropriately labeled as **denial.** The list of problems you will live with (and sometimes die for) in order to continue substance use is amazing.

The degree of psychological dependence is likely to be higher under certain conditions. First, when the drug effect is almost immediate (as occurs with IV drug use), the brain and body are more likely to react with a rapid and intense level of psychological dependence. Second, the more potent the immediate reaction to the drug (as is seen with powerful drugs such as cocaine, amphetamines, and heroin), the more remarkable the psychological dependence is likely to become. Third, the more pleasurable the experience is, the more likely you are to want the drug again.

Physical Dependence

Physical dependence or addiction occurs when the body responds to repeated substance use by building up a level of resistance to the immediate drug effects. In an effort to maintain normal functioning, a variety of changes occur in cell membranes, receptors, and brain chemicals that allow the brain to function normally *despite* the presence of the drug. This process often takes days to weeks to develop. Therefore, it is likely that a similar period of time is required after stopping drug use before physical dependence will diminish or disappear.

So, when you have taken enough of a drug to produce these protective physical changes that make up physical dependence, and then you either cut back in the amount used or stop the drug altogether, a variety of problems known as "withdrawal symptoms" develop. These are often the opposite of what the drug did in the first place, and the symptoms produce a condition known as the **withdrawal or abstinence syndrome.** Simply, these symptoms are the result of the inability of the body in the altered state to function normally unless the drug is present. The re-adaptation of the body to a drug-free environment causes the symptoms that are experienced during drug-withdrawal states.

The good news is that physical addiction or dependence is not seen for all drugs. Only three classes of substances are most likely to be involved here: stimulants (including amphetamine and cocaine), depressants (including alcohol, the Valium-like drugs, and the barbiturates), and opiates (including heroin and most of the prescription pain-killing pills). The withdrawal symptoms seen for the stimulants are the opposite of what is felt with a high, and include sleepiness, an increased appetite, and feelings of depression. The abstinence syndrome observed after stopping depressants includes anxiety, trouble sleeping, a tremor of the hands, and an increased heart rate and body temperature. Finally, the withdrawal syndrome observed with the opiates is characterized by diarrhea, pain in almost all areas of the body including muscles and joints, trouble sleeping, and a runny nose as well as a cough.

It is probably impossible to develop physical dependence on a drug without also having psychological dependence. First, psychological addiction is usually necessary for someone to take the drug in high enough doses over a long enough period of time to develop physical addiction. In addition, once physical dependence occurs, it doesn't take long to learn that it is possible to relieve the pain and discomfort of withdrawal by taking the drug again. This means that restarting the use of depressants or opiates or stimulants is psychologically and physically rewarding. This relief from physical or psychological discomfort is certain to contribute to a high level of psychological dependence.

Tolerance

Actually, it is difficult to discuss physical dependence adequately without bringing up the topic of tolerance. As the body adapts to chronic intake of a drug, especially a brain depressant, a stimulant, or an opiate, the overall effect is that over time the substance produces less intense reactions at the same dose. Another way of describing the same phenomenon is to say that when the drug is taken regularly, it is necessary to increase the doses of the substance to produce the same effects. This change in the body's relationship to the drug is called **tolerance**. The dangers of tolerance include the subsequent need for such high doses that the body's ability to control blood pressure and breathing rate can be severely affected.

Tolerance is the reason why people who drink heavily and regularly can tolerate very high blood alcohol levels and remain relatively awake and alert. Similarly, tolerance is the phenomenon behind the potentially lethal doses of cocaine and amphetamine that the regular user of these drugs can consume without overdosing. However, while the body develops tolerance to some aspects of a drug, it does not produce these changes to all drug actions to an equal degree or at the same rate. This fact becomes very important in cases where an individual increases the amount of drug that he or she is taking to the point that it causes changes in the heartbeat, blood pressure, or the breathing rate significantly enough to threaten life.

As discussed here, it sounds as if tolerance is a relatively straightforward phenomenon. However, there are many different ways that tolerance develops. Some of tolerance comes from the alterations in the body that allow the drug to be broken down or metabolized more quickly (metabolic tolerance). Other forms of tolerance are the result of actual physical changes in the brain or other body organs so that very high blood levels of the drug are required to have major effects (**pharmacodynamic tolerance**). Yet other types of tolerance involve learning how to *appear* to be less impaired through the practice of carrying out actions while high (**behavioral tolerance**). In any event, tolerance is a very important part of the reason why people increase the doses of the drug. Tolerance goes hand-in-hand with physical dependence—although some levels of tolerance can appear without actual physical dependence being present.

A Recap

The drugs of abuse are substances that are fairly easily taken into the body and are rapidly transported to the brain. There, they change brain functioning in predictable ways that, in turn, impact on how you feel. Depending on the route of administration, the dose, the specific drug, and past experiences, every drug discussed in the following chapters is capable of producing psychological dependence. Once this phenomenon has kicked in, the user is willing to spend greater and greater amounts of money and energy and to pay higher and higher prices in physical, social, and interpersonal consequences in order to stay psychologically comfortable. The substances can begin to mean so much psychologically that you can't bring yourself to admit that problems are occurring, that drugs contributed significantly to the difficulties, or that continued use is likely to result in added problems.

Three of the *classes* of drugs (the depressants, stimulants, and opiates—each incorporating perhaps 50 or more specific substances) carry an additional problem. In general, these drugs are so potent and have such strong effects on the brain that in self-defense your brain chemistry is likely to change in a manner that fights against the drug actions. Once this occurs, you are likely to require higher doses of the drug to have the usual effects, a phenomenon known as tolerance. Any time you try to stop taking the drug, symptoms known as the withdrawal syndrome appear, driving you even harder to continue drug use.

This situation develops because the drug offers you feelings that you desire. Obviously, giving up the substances is far from easy because this means saying good-bye to substances that have played an important role in your life. It is almost as if the more that you have invested over the years, the harder it can be to learn to abstain. The next chapter is written in an effort to increase understanding of what these drugs do and why they are at the same time both so attractive and dangerous.

Some Suggested Readings

One of the unique aspects of this book is that, whenever possible, I try to share findings that resulted from research studies. It is relatively infrequently that I will give you my opinion or "clinical impressions." That means that in writing this text, I carried out a thorough literature review from scientific journals and books. My goal was to be as careful as possible that the information you receive is as valid as possible and applies to as broad a range of situations as possible.

As a result of these considerations, the chapters will offer several types of suggested readings. The first is a brief *References* that gives a few of the scientific articles or books directly relevant to the specific chapter. The second, offered at the end of the chapters as *Additional Readings*, is composed of more general books or scientific articles likely to be found in a public library. None of these readings is required in order for you to benefit from this book. However, I am sure that occasionally some readers would benefit from a much broader discussion of some of the things that I present. I also recognize that in some other situations some of you might be a bit skeptical about some of the statements that I make. In either event, you may want to turn to some of the readings that I used in trying to put together this series of chapters.

At the same time, I recognize that this is not a medical textbook. Therefore, I am not giving an extensive list of references for every statement offered. I know that few people will have the time or interest to turn to such a long list of readings. For these reasons, I have focused whenever possible on general review books or articles that might be of help.

Additional Readings*

Gossop, M. *Living with Drugs*, Third Edition. London: Wyldwood House, 1993.

Kandel, D., and Yamaguchi, K. From beer to crack: Developmental patterns in drug involvement. *American Journal of Public Health* 83:851–855, 1993.

Lowinson, J.H., Ruiz, P., Millman, R.B., and Langrod, J.G. (eds.). *Substance Abuse: A Comprehensive Textbook*. Baltimore: Williams and Wilkins, 1997.

Schuckit, M. *Drug and Alcohol Abuse: A Clinical Guide to Diagnosis and Treatment*, Fourth Edition. New York: Plenum Medical Book Company, 1995.

---

*Many readers of this text are not used to the unusual way that articles are referenced in a bibliography. Using the second article as an example, I first list the names of the authors (Kandel and Yamaguchi); I then give the actual title of the article (From beer to crack: Developmental patterns in drug involvement). This is followed by the journal in which the article appeared (the *American Journal of Public Health*). Each major journal is divided into a series of volumes—so 83 is the volume number; and the page numbers (851–855) tell you where to look within that issue or volume of that journal. Finally, the year of publication, 1993, is listed.

Therefore, since 1989, I have published six to ten issues a year of the *Vista Hill Foundation Newsletter*. Because these are very clinically oriented overviews aimed at helping people who are not expert in particular topics to understand more about issues related to drugs, some of these newsletters may be of use to you.

Therefore, in this and in most of the subsequent chapters, I have inserted issues of the *Newsletter* in the Appendix. Regarding Chapter 1, you might turn to the issue entitled:

1. *Chasing the Dragon.*

2

We All Want to Be or Feel
Something Different

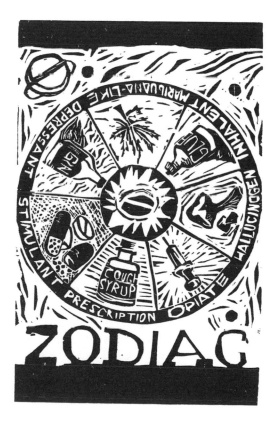

Figure 2.1. The illustration for Chapter 2 is a cross between an emotional and an intellectual message. The huge variety of drugs of abuse that can cause so much turmoil in people's lives actually fall into the seven major categories presented in this zodiac. In Chapter 2, and throughout the text, groups of drugs are divided into the stimulants, depressants, opiates, the marijuana-like drugs or cannabinols, the hallucinogens, the solvents or inhalants, and a miscellaneous category of drugs that includes many prescription and over-the-counter substances. Each slice of the zodiac pie represents an essential graphic design relating to one of the major classes of drugs. Subsequently, within the text when major points regarding a specific drug category are offered, the zodiac sign specific to that group of drugs will be offered in the margin. There, the stimulants, often taken as forms of amphetamines or cocaine, are represented by pills and capsules, the depressants are shown as a bottle of spirits (in this case gin), the leaf of the marijuana plant is given as the representation for cannabinols, hallucinogens are represented by "magic mushrooms," inhalants are signified by a bottle of glue, and the miscellaneous category is represented by a bottle of over-the-counter cough syrup.

Goals

I imagine that few of you have selected this book because you want to become experts in what drugs are and what they do. For most, your goal is likely to be more immediate and practical. It is likely that you are considering the possibility that you might have a problem with some substance, or you are concerned that such a difficulty might exist for someone you care about.

Therefore, this chapter is not written as a text to teach about drugs in general. The goal is to explain enough about what drugs are, what they do, and the ways in which they are similar (as well as dissimilar) in order to help you understand the specific problems you might be facing.

Each type or category of drug offers the chance to "be or feel something different." Some make you feel powerful (stimulants), some make you sedated (depressants), others kill physical pain and cause a floating sensation (opiates), and yet other types of drugs make you mellow (cannabinols), or giddy and confused (solvent inhalants). Many times it is curiosity about these different feeling states that contributes to the decision to "give them a try."

People use a bewildering array of substances. There are probably 250 or more individual drugs available on the streets. This poses a problem for a book like this because there are too many drugs for anyone to learn about in depth. That means that in order for this chapter to work, it is important to develop a way to place the drugs into a limited number of meaningful categories.

A Ph.D. in pharmacology or chemistry would probably choose to group the drugs by their chemical structure. However, most people are interested in what it is that the drugs do to you—how it is that they affect you and the way they make you feel. As a result, the best way to make some sense out of so many substances is by "lumping" things together into groups based on their clinical effects. Therefore, this chapter offers a commonly used scheme to help place the drugs of abuse into some perspective.

Having decided that, another problem develops. One particular drug can have opposite effects at different doses. For example, relatively low levels of cocaine are likely to make people hyperexcited and full of energy, but the same drug at a very high dose could put them into a coma. So, for the purposes of this book, I will **group drugs based on their most prominent effects at the doses at which they are usually taken.**

As luck would have it, grouping substances this way is an excellent predictor of the pattern of problems they are likely to cause. The 250 or so drugs can be fairly simply divided into categories based on how, at the usual doses taken, they make you feel and their other prominent effects.

This chapter describes a series of substances that fall roughly into the categories listed below. These groups and some examples of each are outlined in Table 2.1. Then, Table 2.2 outlines some

Table 2.1
Classes or Groups of Drugs Likely to Be Abused

Drug group	Examples
Stimulants[a]	All forms of amphetamines, all forms of cocaine, all prescription diet pills
Depressants[a]	Alcohol, almost all antianxiety drugs (such as Valium), all prescription sleeping pills
Opiates[a]	Almost all prescription pain pills (such as Darvon, Percodan), codeine, demerol, heroin, methodone
Cannabinols	All forms of marijuana
Hallucinogens	LSD, "magic mushrooms," MDMA (ecstasy), mescaline, peyote, psilocybin
Solvents or Inhalants	Acetone, aerosol gases (hydrocarbons), benzene, ether, gasoline, glue, paint thinner, toluene, whiteout
Others	Amyl and butyl nitrite (poppers), nitrous oxide (laughing gas), phencyclidine (PCP)

[a]These three classes of drugs are capable of producing physical addiction and can cause withdrawal symptoms when a user stops taking them.

of the street names for each important group. The following are the categories of drugs we will consider:

1. The *stimulants* (like amphetamines, cocaine, and weight-reducing pills), drugs that, at the usual doses taken, make you feel powerful, alert, and stimulated.
2. The *depressants* (including alcohol, the Valium-type drugs, and all barbiturates), drugs that usually make you feel sedated and tired.
3. The *opiates* (heroin, codeine, methadone, and almost all prescription pain pills), drugs that make you feel no pain.
4. The *cannabinols* (marijuana, hashish, charas, ganja, and bhang), drugs that make you feel mellow.
5. The *hallucinogens* (such as LSD, mescaline, peyote, psilocybin, and "magic mushrooms"), drugs that intensify perceptions of the senses.
6. The *solvents* or *inhalants* (including glue and aerosols), drugs that make you feel giddy and confused.
7. I have also developed a "miscellaneous" or "other" category for drugs that are capable of causing problems but that do not naturally fall into one of these six categories. Drugs discussed in this seventh category include amyl and butyl nitrite ("poppers"), various over-the-counter drugs, and caffeine and nicotine.

For each major type of substance, I will describe the intoxication or prominent effects, give a bit of its history, and present a brief outline of the usual course of events associated with its use. I have set off the groups by subheadings based on how each drug makes a user feel to make it easier to find your way to the substances of greatest concern to you.

As part of the discussion of each drug, I touch a bit on the pattern of use in the general population. However, there is a general property of use that can be briefly presented here. In the course of experimentation with different drugs, people usually begin with the most widely available substances and then move on through the agents less available (or less acceptable to society).

Table 2.2
A Brief List of "Street" Drug Names

CNS depressants[a]

Amies	Double trouble	Peanuts	Sleepers
Blue birds	Downers	Peter (chloral hydrate)	Soapers
Blue devil	Downs	Quads	T-bird
Blue heaven	Goofballs	Rainbows	Tooies
Blues	Green and whites (Librium)	Red birds	Toolies
Bullets	Greenies	Red devils	Tranqs (Librium-type)
Candy	Ludes	Roaches (Librium)[b]	Wallbangers
Christmas trees	Nebbies	Seccy	Yellow jackets
Dolls	Nembles	Seggy	Yellows

Stimulants

Amphetamines

Bennies	Double cross	Pink and green
Blue angels	Footballs	Roses
Blue beauties	Green and clears	Speed
Chris	Greenies	Speedball (heroin plus cocaine)
Christine	Hearts	Truck drivers
Christmas tree	L.A. turnarounds	Turnarounds
Coast to coast	Lip poppers	Uppers
Copilot	Meth	Ups
Crisscross	Oranges	Wake-ups
Crossroads	Peaches	Whites
Crystal (IV methamphetamine)[b]	Pep pills	Yellow jackets
	Pinks	

Cocaine

Blow	Lady
C	Nose
Coke	Nose candy
Crack	Rock
Dust	Snow
Dynamite	Speedball
Flake	Toot
Gold dust	White
Heaven dust	

Opiates

Heroin		Other	
Bomb	Horse	Black (opium)	PG or PO (paregoric)
Brother	Junk	Blue velvet (paregoric plus	Pinks and grays (Darvon)
Brown	Mexican Mud	antihistamine)	Poppy (opium)
Cat	Scat	Dollies (methadone)[b]	Tar (opium)
Chinese white	Shit	M (morphine)	Terp (terpin hydrate or
Dogie	Skag	Microdots (morphine)	cough syrup with
Duji	Smack	Miss Emma (morphine)	codeine)
Duster (cigarette)	Snow	Morphy (morphine)	T's and blues (Talwin and
H	Stuff	O (opium)	antihistamine)
H and stuff	Tango and cash	Pellets (opium)	

Cannabinols

Marijuana			Hashish-like (more potent)	
Acapulco gold	Grass	Locoweed	Sativa	Bhang	Hash
Afghani	Hay	Mary Jane	Stick	Charas	Rope
A stick	Hemp	Mexican	Stuff	Gage	Sweet Lucy
Boo	J	MJ	Tea	Ganja	THC
Bomb	Jane	Muggles	Texas tea		
Brick	Jive	Pot	Thai sticks		
Buddha sticks	Joint	Reefer	Weed		
Columbian	Key or kee	Roach[b]	Yesca		
Gold	Lid				

29

Table 2.2
(Continued)

Phencyclidine (PCP)

Angel	Criptal	Hog	Mist	Shermans	Supergrass
Aurora	Dummy mist	Jet	Mumm dust	Sherms	Superjoint
Bust bee	Goon	K	Peace pill	Special L.A. coke	Trangs
Cheap cocaine	Green	Lovely	Purple	Superacid	Tranq
Cosmos	Guerrilla	Mauve	Rocket fuel	Supercoke	Whack

Hallucinogens

Acid (LSD)	Crystal[b]	Love drug (MDMA)	Mescal (mescaline)	Pearly gates (morning glory seeds)
Blue dots (LSD)	Cube (LSD)	Lysergide (LSD)	Mexican mushroom (psilocybin)	
Blue heaven (LSD)	D (LSD)	Magic Mushroom (psilocybin)	Microdots (LSD)	Sugar (LSD)
Buttons (peyote)	Deaths head (mushroom)	Mellow drug of America (MDA)	Mushroom (psilocybin)	White lightning (LSD)
Cactus (mescaline)	Hevenly blue (LSD)	Mesc (mescaline)	Owsleys (LSD)	25 (LSD)

[a]Moderate length of action *like* secobarbital unless otherwise noted.
[b]Many drugs have the same name.

Therefore, most people are likely to begin with caffeine and nicotine and move on quickly to alcohol. If they go further, the next drug likely to be experienced is marijuana in any of its forms, meaning that almost everyone who tries marijuana has had some experience with caffeine, nicotine, and alcohol. If the person decides to go beyond marijuana, he or she is likely to experiment with any one drug or combination of stimulants (such as cocaine or amphetamine), depressants (such as the Valium-type drugs), or hallucinogens. The more often these are used and the higher the doses of these drugs that are taken, the greater the likelihood that the person involved is taking other substances as well. Only a small percentage of users are likely to progress to opiate-type drugs (such as heroin) or IV use of any of the other drugs. So, whereas each drug is described as if it exists in isolation, it usually should be viewed as part of a more complex picture.

The Stimulants: The Drugs That (at First) Make You Feel Happy (Powerful, Alert, and Stimulated)

What the Stimulants Are (Including Amphetamines, Cocaine, Methylphenidate, or Ritalin, and Weight-Reducing Pills) and How They Are Used

These drugs, capable of producing physical addiction, are appropriately named as stimulants because their most prominent actions at the usual doses are to give feelings of energy, happiness, power, a decreased desire for sleep, and a diminished appetite. The drugs include every form of amphetamine (such as benzedrine, dexedrine, and methamphetamine), every form of cocaine (from coca paste, to cocaine powder, to freebase, to crack or rock), and, as far as I know, every prescription diet pill. Technically, this group of substances also includes caffeine and nicotine, but because these two are legal for adults and much less powerful in their immediate effects, my emphasis will be placed on the more potent drugs.

Regarding cocaine, the major difference between freebase cocaine and cocaine powder (cocaine hydrochloride) is the temperature at which they melt. Because of its lower melting point, freebase is able to be smoked, whereas the powder, with a higher temperature needed before it goes up in smoke, is usually snorted. Crack and rock (the same substance with different names on the two coasts of the United States) were also developed with low melting points in mind so that they could be smoked, but they were mostly produced in this form as a "marketing" tool rather than a new and entirely different form of the drug. Although amphetamine highs last longer than those from cocaine, most clinicians believe that those who use cocaine heavily cannot tell when they have been given an injection of amphetamine as a substitute, and those who use amphetamine heavily can easily be fooled by cocaine. It is not surprising, therefore, that the problem pattern associated with both types of drugs is quite similar. The diet-type pills share the whole profile of problems of stimulants, including subsequent mood swings and nervousness.

Most people who try amphetamines or cocaine (and perhaps 20% to 40% of young adult Americans do) discover that it is difficult to stop taking the substance during a particular evening. A small percentage keep returning to the drug and soon increase their use to multiple times per day. It is for this 10% or so of the cocaine-using population that a "run" or binge of stimulant use is likely to occur. This involves increasing doses, subsequent exhaustion, and a high probability of developing severe suspiciousness and the hearing of voices (auditory hallucinations). The run is likely to end only when the supply runs out, when the user becomes exhausted, or if a crisis results in arrest or hospitalization. When he or she stops, the user is then likely to experience a period of days of intense depression followed by many weeks of mood swings. Unfortunately, such a user is likely to seek out new supplies of the drug in order to stop these bad feelings.

Their History

The use and abuse of stimulants date back many centuries, probably occurring even before the natives of the Andes Mountains in South America discovered that chewing coca leaves could decrease hunger and fatigue. Cocaine was first identified scientifically in the mid-1800s, and amphetamines were first artificially produced later in that century. It seems as if whenever these drugs (especially amphetamines and cocaine) become plentiful, there is an epidemic of severe problems. At least one such epidemic occurred in Germany following World War I, with a similar problem in Japan following World War II. In both instances, the rate of violence and of psychiatric symptoms such as hallucinations seemed to have increased.

The more recent surge of stimulant use, especially cocaine, in the United States has had a major impact on both business and law enforcement. It has been estimated that in the 1980s the street value of the cocaine sold approached 32 billion U.S. dollars per year (1). If true, that would place the "business" of cocaine well within the top ten U.S. "companies." Similarly, cocaine production, processing, and distribution have become major components of the economies of a number of Central and South American countries.

The flow of this much money has spawned huge problems for society. Even setting aside the impact on emergency room visits and lost work days, society's response to this illegal traffic in drugs has clogged both the courts and the prisons. Few other influences have so severely tested a nation's values and resources as have these drugs.

In summary, the stimulants are a group of very powerful drugs. They produce immediate intoxication, are likely to lead to strong feelings of psychological dependence, and are also capable of producing physical addiction. Many people in the drug abuse field consider this group of substances as one of the most dangerous and difficult to control of the drugs of abuse.

The Depressants: Drugs That (at First) Make You "High" (Sedated and Tired)

What the Depressants (Alcohol, All Valium-type Drugs, All Barbiturates Such as Seconal, Miltown, or Equanil) Are and How They Are Used

Because 90% of people in the United States drink at some time during their lives, and perhaps half of drinkers have some temporary alcohol-related difficulties, problems with depressants are the most common of the substance abuse difficulties of the Western world. The other brain depressants, including the barbiturates and the Valium-type drugs, are among the most commonly prescribed medications, with an estimated 15% of American adults having used these drugs during any year (2). Somewhere between 5% and 10% of the population has taken depressant medications, often on prescription, for at least a month at a time, indicating that a fair number of people are likely to have developed some level of psychological dependence on depressants other than alcohol (3). All of the brain depressants are capable of producing physical dependence.

The effects of alcohol and the other depressants when taken for a "high" are remarkably similar. These drugs are usually ingested orally, reaching a peak level in the bloodstream within ten to thirty minutes. When the drug is building up in the blood (and blood levels are rising), most people report feeling more relaxed, a bit sleepy, and are likely to have some problems thinking clearly. At the same time, some level of incoordination is likely to occur. When blood levels of depressants are decreasing, most people experience feelings of sleepiness and irritability and continue to have some level of problems in thinking clearly.

The usual course of problems with alcohol serves as a good illustration of what typically occurs during use of a depressant drug. Because alcohol is both relatively inexpensive and also one of the most powerful of the legal substances, it is often seen by children as a badge of maturity. Therefore, the first experience with alcohol (other than taking a sip of a parent's drink) is likely to occur between the ages of twelve and fourteen years. The first time enough alcohol is taken to cause some level of intoxication is likely to occur in the midteens, and somewhere between sixteen and twenty years of age, many drinkers have their first temporary life problem from alcohol. These problems include skipping school or work in order to "party" or because of a hangover, drinking so much during an evening that they forget part of what went on (a blackout), and driving while impaired with alcohol (even if no accident or arrest occurred). Fortunately, most drinkers learn how to control alcohol intake by their mid- to late twenties so that heavy drinking and even temporary problems are likely to disappear.

However, by the late teens to midthirties, the people who are developing alcoholism (alcohol abuse or dependence) differ from this usual story in important ways. This person finds it increasingly difficult to refrain from consistently consuming large amounts of alcohol, despite making his or her best efforts to do so. One of the most characteristic behaviors of the problem drinker is the way he or she will alternate periods of abstinence with times during which large amounts of alcohol are consumed. Another characteristic behavior is temporary controlled drinking, when the user successfully (but temporarily) limits his or her intake of alcohol to a certain number of drinks per day or a few days per week. These behaviors represent the problem drinker's attempt to establish control over his or her alcohol intake. However, attempts to establish periods of limited alcohol consumption almost invariably fail, and the user is likely to experience repeated patterns of alcohol-related problems over the years. Despite these difficulties, and despite the best efforts of the user to abstain or limit alcohol consumption, any subsequent use of the drug increases the chance of severe problems.

Much less is known about the pattern of problems associated with abuse of barbiturates and Valium-type drugs. Some people begin their experimentation with these substances in a party situation or in an attempt to try a different type of "high." A large group of those who develop difficulties with these drugs, however, begin taking them on prescription and escalate the doses on their own. From either starting point, what is likely to occur is an escalation of intake, the development of psychological dependence that makes it difficult to give up the drug despite the best intentions, the possible development of physical dependence that makes it even harder to stop, and a typical off-again on-again course of problems.

History of Depressant-type Drugs

Depressant-type drugs have been available since Biblical times (and before). People quickly discovered that fruits and grains allowed to rot in tepid water, especially in the presence of sugar, produced a fluid that could be pleasant to the taste and cause feelings of intoxication. This discovery was the beginning of a long and complex line of drug use and abuse that has altered history. Repeated depressant intoxication contributed to the debauchery and downfall of the Roman Empire, and it has affected the outcome of most wars where intoxicated soldiers were likely to have diminished abilities to fight.

The modern era of potent depressant-type medications probably began in the mid-1800s with the production of barbiturates. These early medications were widely prescribed for a variety of neurological, medical, and emotional problems. However, these substances suffered from a number of severe drawbacks, including ability to cause death at high doses, and, at even lower doses, an ability to diminish appropriate body functioning (including decreasing heartbeat, blood pressure, and breathing rate). These drugs were also capable of causing severe intoxication and of predisposing people who used them toward psychological and physical dependence.

Because of these problems, the world welcomed what turned out to be only slightly safer forms of depressant-type drugs in the 1950s. These new substances came in the form of the "minor tranquilizer" meprobamate, which was marketed as Equanil and

Miltown. The discovery that this drug also had many of the problems associated with barbiturates helped spur on the search for "safer" depressant-type drugs, leading to the development of the Valium-type substances (also called benzodiazepines). Although an improvement because of the lower levels of problems likely to be seen if the medications are taken exactly as prescribed, these newer depressants share the dangers of the production of dependence and a potential for overdose deaths when higher doses are used.

In summary, the depressants include a wide range of prescription drugs (the Valium-like benzodiazepines as well as the barbiturates) and alcohol. As a result, they contain both useful prescribed drugs and the most widely abused substances.

The Opiates: Drugs That Make You Feel No Pain (and Nod Off or Float)

What the Opiates Are (Heroin, Codeine, Methadone, and Almost All Prescription Pain Pills) and How They Are Used

The opiates consist of a group of physically addicting drugs that at the usual doses markedly decrease feelings of physical pain while causing only modest levels of sedation. They include all of the substances that come from the opium poppy plant, such as opium, heroin, morphine, and codeine. In addition, almost all of the prescription pain killers, when taken in high enough doses, can cause the same type of intoxication and produce the same pattern of problems as heroin. These prescription drugs include Dilaudid (hydromorphone), Percodan (oxycodone), Demerol (meperidine), Talwin (pentazocine), and less potent medications such as Darvon (propoxyphene).

Each of these drugs produces feelings of moderate drowsiness, changes in mood, and, at very high doses, can cause death. At the usual doses taken for a "high," there is a floating feeling, euphoria, and a series of physical changes. These changes include a decreased rate of breathing, a slowing down of the spontaneous movements of the intestine (causing constipation), a decrease in the size of the pupil of the eye, and, for some people, a tremor of the hands and some twitching of the muscles. When taken by any route of administration in high doses, but especially likely when taken IV, these drugs can cause severe slowing of breathing and heart rates resulting in death by overdose.

Perhaps 10% of adolescents have ever used opiates for a "high" (4). However, only 1% to 3% of the population have consistently demonstrated severe psychological and physical addiction to the opiates (4). The number of opiate users can sometimes temporarily double when street supplies of opiates such as heroin become particularly plentiful or cheap.

There are at least two major roads to psychological and physical addiction with opiates. The first is medical. Some men and women become addicted in medical settings, a situation most likely to develop in people who take the drugs for chronic pain syndromes. Another type of "medical" addiction is evidenced by the increased rate of problems with these drugs among health care professionals, especially physicians and nurses.

However, the majority of people who develop problems with opiates began use of these substances through the second road to addiction, a "social" setting. The first use of an opiate is likely to occur rather late in the continuum of drug use after alcohol, the marijuana-type drugs, and after some experimentation with other depressants and stimulants. The first use of heroin, for example, is likely to be seen in the late teens (probably an average of about 18 years), with several years of "experimentation" usually occurring before severe problems appear. Psychological dependence is likely to occur early in the course of experimentation with these drugs and is usually first experienced in the early twenties. Physical dependence includes an obvious withdrawal syndrome when substance use stops and is often seen a few years later than psychological addiction.

As is true with all of the drug-related lifestyles, when you continue use of the substance, you put yourself at a huge risk for severe illness and early death. In order to avoid physical withdrawal, IV users of heroin have to "shoot up" every four to six or so hours, making it almost impossible to hold a regular job. This means that many street users get money for these expensive drugs by stealing, prostitution, or committing other crimes. Often, heavy users are first arrested in the late teens to early twenties. One study following a group of heroin addicts over time reported that more than 25% of the group died over a twenty-year period (5). Causes of death included suicide (related to the severe mood swings that can occur), being killed by the police or in a drug-related violent incident, accidents, and infectious diseases associated with the use of IV drugs (including AIDS). Since as many as 80% of IV drug users have been found to be carrying the AIDS virus in San Francisco, the rate of early death has probably increased remarkably in recent years (6).

Their History

As is true for the stimulants and the depressants, the opiates have been around for a very long time. Indeed, many of the pain-killing effects of home medicines in the Middle Ages were related to opium-like properties. The widespread use of opiates in Europe and the United States was first documented in the late 1800s. This wave of use created widespread abuse and psychological as well as physical dependence that was largely the result of how cheap and highly available these drugs were in over-the-counter medicines. Interestingly, this epidemic of addiction was observed to affect mostly middle-class women via over-the-counter or prescribed medications, a condition that continued until these drugs were placed under legal control in the United States in the early 1900s.

Since that time, as a consequence of the Harrison Act that required a doctor's prescription to obtain these substances, legal access to opiates has been kept relatively limited. However, this altered pattern of availability did not cause these drugs to disappear but, rather, forced them into an "underground" that simmered beneath the surface for decades. There was an increase in "street" use of these substances in the United States following World War II and a virtual explosion of use during the Vietnam War. Soldiers, many of whom had no experience with opiate-like agents, were sent far from home, placed under great stress, and lived in a country where opium was cheap and easily available. A substantial minority (estimated by some to be as high as a third) of soldiers "in country" experimented with these drugs, usually through smoking. One of the common mechanisms for taking the drug was "chasing the dragon," where opium is heated on a piece of tin foil, and the subsequent smoke is directly inhaled. Fortunately, most men who began use of opiates in this very unusual environment did not continue their use of the substance once they returned home. On the other hand, soldiers who had had experience with either IV drugs or who had used opiates on the street before going to Vietnam were quite likely to find themselves repeatedly using these substances once they returned to the United States.

A small but persistent proportion of the general population continue to use these drugs on the "streets." Interestingly, this usage has tended to expand and contract in an epidemic pattern, depending upon the cost and overall availability of substances like heroin. One example of this phenomenon occurred in the 1960s, when a large number of overdose deaths and other opium-related problems were noted in New York following a huge shipment of inexpensive opiates into the city.

In summary, the opiates are a group of drugs that consist of all of the direct products of the poppy plant and almost all prescription painkillers. Depending on the dose, all of these drugs cause a similar high, all are capable of producing physical as well as psychological dependence, and the withdrawal syndrome from one drug of this class looks quite similar to that from any other. Most users begin with occasional experimentation that escalates to regular intake after a period of some months or a couple of years. Once problems begin, especially after IV drug use has entered the picture, stopping drugs becomes a life or death decision.

Forms of Marijuana: Drugs That Make You Feel Mellow

What the Cannabinols Are (Marijuana, Hashish, Charas, Ganja, Bhang) and How They Are Used

The cannabinols or marijuana-type drugs all contain the same active ingredient, delta-9-tetrahydrocannabinol (abbreviated as THC). The specific name of the type of cannabinol depends upon the part of the marijuana plant from which it comes. Hashish and charas are produced from the resin of the flowering tops, bhang from the less potent dried leaves and flowers, ganja from the resin of small leaves; most of the marijuana in the United States is produced from the leaves themselves.Usually inhaled as smoke, but also taken by eating (which causes a slower onset but a more long-lasting high), the drug effects are quite similar. At the usual doses, people experience euphoria, a floating or mellow feeling, along with a perception that the passage of time has slowed down. Most users also note an increase in appetite. At very high doses, people can become agitated and confused and might have hallucinations, especially seeing flashing lights or geometrical shapes.

The intoxication is also associated with some undesirable effects. These include a slowing of decision-making and reaction times (which can interfere with driving abilities), an impaired ability to think clearly (which can last for several days and interfere with school and work performance), some mild feelings of suspiciousness and paranoia, a mild tremor or shaking of the hands, a dry mouth, and bloodshot eyes. The interference with judgment and driving ability along with the potential medical problems are among the major dangers for these drugs, as you will see in Chapter 3.

The marijuana-type drugs have been tried on at least one occasion by as many as 60 million Americans and are the most commonly used "street" drugs. The average person's first use of marijuana usually takes place in the mid- to late teens. Forty percent to 60% of high school seniors have tried this drug, and 5% to 7% use marijuana daily (4).

As is true with all of the drugs discussed here, the greater the amount of marijuana used, the greater the chance that other drugs are also being taken fairly regularly, including alcohol, depressants, and stimulants. There is also an association between use of any of the cannabinol-type drugs and the experience of other life problems, including difficulties within the home and at school.

Their History

Cannabinol is truly an ancient drug with evidence of use almost three thousand years before the birth of Christ. Prior to the turn of the 20th century, it was most often taken in the Middle East and Orient in a variety of forms, especially as hashish, charas, bhang, and ganja. Use of marijuana-type agents, mostly as marijuana tobacco and hashish, was observed in the 1940s in the United States in a small but substantial group of people, especially those living in relatively poor inner-city areas, but use patterns exploded in the late 1950s to the mid-1960s. At that point, growth of the plant in the United States, along with a massive expansion of imports from other areas of the world, resulted in a marked increase in the number of people who have had experience with these drugs. The proportion of users continued to increase throughout the 1960s, reaching all strata of society. As discussed above, this drug is now one of the most common substances of abuse.

Although the major use is on the "streets" to obtain a high, the drug does have some medicinal properties. For example, marijuana has been found to relieve some types of severe eye pressure (narrow angle of glaucoma) and is also used by some cancer patients to minimize the nausea and vomiting following chemotherapy.

In summary, the cannabinols actually represent a single drug that is taken in different forms that differ mostly in their potency. These substances are truly ancient, were taken by a small proportion of the population in the United States in the 1940s and 1950s, and experienced escalated use by the 1960s to the point that almost 60% of young Americans in most major urban areas have had experience with this drug (4). The intoxication with marijuana products is relatively mild, but there are significant health dangers associated with its use. Intoxication can also impair driving abilities and, thus, contribute to accidents.

Hallucinogens: Drugs That Intensify Perceived Senses

What the Hallucinogens Are (LSD, Mescaline, Peyote, Psilocybin, "Magic Mushrooms," MDMA or Ecstasy) and How They Are Used

The hallucinogens are a group of diverse drugs that all share the ability at the usual doses to produce a sensation of intensi- fied feelings and perceptions. These include heightened perceptions of the impact of colors, sounds, and touches. At higher doses, intoxication can include hallucinations of lights, colors, and geometrical figures, but hallucinations that focus on people or events are more rare. Surprisingly, the person usually knows that what he or she is seeing is a result of the drug, or, in other words, the individual usually has insight into the experience. Many of these substances are related to amphetamines and, therefore, also cause feelings of excitement and increased energy.

In addition, there are a variety of street drugs that, although not true hallucinogens, tend to be used by people for the stimulation and increased feelings of ability to perceive senses that they cause. Probably the most prominent of these drugs is **phencyclidine** or PCP, which at the usual clinical doses (about 10 milligrams) mimics many of the effects of hallucinogens. However, PCP at only slightly higher doses can cause severe confusion and agitation, a combination that can often result in violence. Unfortunately, in distinction from what is usually observed with almost all other drugs mentioned in this book, this severe level of confusion with PCP can last for two or three months at a time.

Other drugs that can be used for an effect with some similarity to hallucinogens include **laughing gas** (nitrous oxide), and **morning glory seeds.** The length of drug effects differs depending upon the specific drug used. For example, LSD produces an onset of feelings within a half-hour to an hour, a peak effect at about ninety minutes, with some lingering intoxication observed for as long as six to twelve hours. Most other hallucinogens produce changes that last between two and eight hours.

This type of drug did not become popular on the "street" until the 1960s, when use increased dramatically. Research indicates that the peak years of use of these substances was in the late 1960s to early 1970s, with a subsequent leveling off and decrease (7). However, even in the 1980s, almost 25% of people in the eighteen- to twenty-five-year range had used a hallucinogen at some time in their lives, with figures that have ranged from about 15% to 25% ever since.

Their History

These drugs are hardly new. Many of the substances, peyote for example, have been administered as part of religious ceremonies and social gatherings by Native American groups for 2,000 years or more. Some are still incorporated into forms of religious rites.

As described above, experimentation with hallucinogens in most Western countries greatly expanded during the "drug explosion" of the early to mid-1960s. Hallucinogens became identified in many people's minds with the "hippie generation," where the drugs were used as a group experience, especially at folk and rock concerts. At the same time, however, because hallucinogens such as LSD are associated with feelings of increased intensities of sensory perceptions, in the early 1960s, some psychotherapists experimented with the potential use of these drugs to help patients expand their feeling states and "get in touch with" their innermost thoughts. Unfortunately, all research efforts demonstrated no benefit to any user in the context of psychotherapy, and the drug fell out of favor in clinical settings. Despite these data, twenty to thirty years later another hallucinogen (Ecstasy or MDMA) was touted for identical possible clinical properties with similar results—no evidence that these drugs enhance any therapeutic efforts.

In summary, the hallucinogens do not usually produce hallucinations. Their most prominent effect is a feeling of increased sensory perceptions. When hallucinations occur they are usually visual, often involve colors or shapes, and the person almost always recognizes that the things that he or she are seeing are caused by the drug.

The Solvents or Inhalants: Drugs That Make You Feel as if You Are Floating and That Cause Confusion

What the Solvents Are and How They Are Used

The glues, solvents, aerosols, and other inhalants include a broad range of substances that are all taken into the body through the lungs (inhalation) to cause a rapid onset of giddiness and lightheadedness. Every one of these substances is capable of interfering with the functioning of cells in the body that contain fat in their skins or membranes, including brain cells. Therefore, their use is likely to interfere with cell membrane functioning, which will cause alterations in how efficiently the cell functions and decrease the ability of the brain to carry out its work. Although those changes are usually temporary, with prolonged heavy use, the brain damage can be permanent. Heavy use can also cause damage to the heart, liver, and kidneys. The solvents include glues (containing toluene, benzene, chloroform, and other substances), the contents of some aerosol cans (usually fluorinated hydrocarbons or freon), nail polish removers (often containing acetone), paint thinners (with toluene, acetone, naphtha, and methanol), and gasoline products (containing gasoline, toluene, benzene, and petroleum ether).

These are usually among the first substances that teenagers try for a "high." Because use is associated with headache, nausea, and the variety of medical problems described in the next chapter, and because the high is not very sophisticated—just confusion—most people stop using these agents after a few tries. Only a small percentage of people (probably less than 1% of the general population) continue to use these substances in adulthood, whereas the majority of the 20% to 30% of adolescents who have tried these drugs decide that they are not worth pursuing any further. Teenagers in rural settings as well as men and women in prisons are the most likely to continue the use of solvents.

Their History

There are reports of intermittent use of solvents to cause a high that date back over a hundred years. More widespread use, however, probably began in the early 1960s. Despite efforts of manufacturers to modify products like paints and glues to make them less likely to be abused, the use of this type of agent has continued.

In summary, solvents cause a fairly simple and direct (although dangerous) feeling of giddiness and lightheadedness. Although a significant proportion of young men and women have experimented with this type of drug, continued use into adulthood is not common.

Drugs That Make You Feel—Well, Almost Anything

 If a substance can find its way into the body, is transported by the blood to the brain, and changes how a person feels, and if the use doesn't cause immediate intense sickness, someone will abuse it. Therefore, this section could deal with any prescription, over-the-counter, or street drug that produces some form of mental change. To be realistic, however, I have chosen to focus on a few drugs that don't obviously fall into any of the other categories but that might pose problems for some of the people reading this text.

Amyl and butyl nitrite ("poppers") are used as a prescription drug for heart problems. These drugs are inhaled after breaking or popping a glass vial (that's where the street name came from), or can be taken as a gas obtained from adult sex stores where it is sold as "rush," "kick," and "belt," among other names. Although it could have been discussed with the solvents, such as glue, the actual feelings people get with the nitrites are different enough that I've chosen to discuss them separately. Inhaling the vapors of any of these gasses produces a feeling of fullness in the head (probably relating to a temporary enlargement of some of the blood vessels in the brain), a mild euphoria, a perception that time has slowed down, and possibly some increase in sexual feelings or libido. These effects come on in minutes and can last for as long as a quarter of an hour. The drugs are also thought to cause relaxation of body muscles (which might enhance sexual enjoyment). The average user is in his late teens to early twenties, where perhaps 15% have had some experience with the drug, with a much higher rate of repeated intake among homosexuals (perhaps 60%) (4). The nitrite inhalants are most likely to be used by men, individuals with a high number of sexual partners, and heavy drinkers. In addition to psychological dependence, the difficulties associated with nitrite inhalants include impairment of the body's ability to fight off infections (immune functioning problems), a bronchitis-like syndrome, and a possible increased risk for various types of cancers.

There are a variety of **over-the-counter (OTC)** drugs that can be abused. These are discussed in much more detail in my 1995 text for professionals, listed in the Suggested Readings. The drugs include medications that can cause sleepiness (for example, antihistamines that are used in OTC sleeping pills and antianxiety drugs such as Sominex and Compoz), nose sprays and pills used to treat nasal congestion (which, in high doses can cause a speeded up feeling similar to the stimulants), and some of the OTC cough medicines that contain alcohol in concentrations as high as 50 proof (25%) as well as opiate-like anticough components such as dextromethorphan that resemble weak forms of codeine.

Whereas each of these types of drugs causes some sort of prominent psychological change, it is less obvious why some people abuse other OTC pain pills such as aspirin, phenacetin, acetaminophen, and ibuprofen. Chronic intake of these drugs can cause stomach ulcers, liver failure, and kidney destruction, but despite these dangers, some people develop a psychological dependence, feeling that they cannot make it through the day without taking these drugs on a regular basis. Similarly, the various forms of OTC laxatives are capable of producing psychological dependence in people who fear that they cannot move their bowels regularly without them, despite the dangers of vitamin deficiencies, muscle weakness, and excessive loss of body water that can occur with prolonged use of laxatives.

It is important, in a book of this sort, to pay adequate attention to the two most commonly abused legal drugs, **caffeine** and **nicotine**. It is obvious that many people develop psychological dependence on coffee and other caffeinated beverages, and some even feel as if they must take over-the-counter caffeine products regularly (such as No-Doz—a substance that contains 100 milligrams of caffeine, about the amount found in a medium-strength cup of coffee). There is also evidence that some people who regularly take caffeine develop a syndrome of headache, sweating, and feeling as if they can't think straight for several days when they try to cut down on their coffee intake—a condition that resembles a mild withdrawal syndrome. This seems to indicate a form of physical addiction in at least some people.

Even more intense and obvious levels of psychological and physical dependence develop with nicotine. This pattern of problems is impressive when you consider the fact that 28% of Americans still choose to continue to smoke (with a similar percentage of new users choosing to begin this practice each year (8). They do so despite all of the evidence that these substances increase the risk for cancer, heart disease, problems in blood circulation, and impair optimal development of the fetus in the womb. Although the average person reading this book is probably not primarily concerned about these types of drugs, it doesn't hurt to point out that issues of psychological and physical dependence can develop, problem patterns often are seen, and the stages of recovery described in this book have some applications to these less potent but very important substances.

A Recap

All drugs that cause problems of abuse and dependence share a number of characteristics. They are all taken into the body fairly easily, all find their way to the brain fairly quickly, and all change how the user feels emotionally. A solid proportion of the drugs that are abused on the street produce feelings of energy and powerfulness (the stimulants), another thirty or so drugs act by decreasing feelings of anxiety and slowing down general brain functioning (the depressants), whereas still others cause a milder level of sedation but are very powerful in killing physical pain (the opiates). These three categories of drugs not only produce psychological dependence, but they are also difficult to stop because of the physical addiction or dependence that can develop. Other categories of drugs offer a "laid back" and floating feeling (the cannabinols), increase the intensity of the perception of the senses (the hallucinogens and PCP), or cause a short-lived, giddy and confused state (the solvents and inhalants).

But each of these substances, as well as the miscellaneous drugs briefly described above, is capable of producing a condition where the drug itself means more to the person than the problems it is causing. When this happens, people are usually reluctant to admit that they have life problems, are resistant to the idea that the substances caused the problems or at least made them worse, or refuse to believe that they are having trouble controlling substance intake (no matter how many times they have failed at long-term abstinence or attempts at controlled use in the past). This process of denial, seen for all of these substances, makes sense because without it few people would continue substance use after the problems developed. This chapter is entitled "We All Want to Be or Feel Something Different." Some want to be someone or something they are not. It is in this context that you might begin to take drugs because you like the feelings of happiness, sedation, floating sensations, and so on. Each of you begins the use of these substances absolutely convinced that you will only experiment for a period of time—just to change the feeling, or give the thrill for a few moments, or for an afternoon or evening. Few people are likely to be aware of the dangers that are likely to develop from the search for new and different "feelings." Those potential problems are discussed in more detail in Chapter 3.

References

1. Gawin, F. H., and Ellinwood, E. H., Jr. Cocaine and other stimulants: Actions, abuse, and treatment. *New England Journal of Medicine* 318: 1173–1182, 1988.
2. Busto, U. Patterns of benzodiazepine abuse and dependence. *British Journal of Addictions* 81:87–94, 1986.
3. Chaplin, S. Benzodiazepine prescribing. *Lancet* 1:120–121, 1988.
4. Jaffe, J. H. Drug addiction and drug abuse. In Gilman, A. G., Goodman, L. S., Rall, T. W., Murad, F. (Eds) *The Pharmacological Basis of Therapeutics,* Seventh Edition. New York: MacMillan, 1985, pp. 532–581.
5. Vaillant, G. E. A 20-year follow-up of New York narcotic addicts. *Archives of General Psychiatry* 29:237–241, 1973.
6. Friedland, G. H., and Klein, R. S. Transmission of the human immunodeficiency virus. *New England Journal of Medicine* 317:1125–1135, 1987.
7. Schuckit, M. A. *Drug and Alcohol Abuse: A Clinical Guide to Diagnosis and Treatment,* Fourth Edition. New York: Plenum, 1995.
8. Fielding, J. E. Smoking: Health effects and control. *New England Journal of Medicine* 313:491–498, 1985.

Additional Readings

Gold, M. S. Cocaine (and crack): Clinical aspects. In: Lowinson, J. H., Ruiz, P., Millman, R. B., and Langrod, J. G. *Substance Abuse: A Comprehensive Textbook*, Second Edition. Baltimore: Williams & Wilkins, 1997, pp. 181–198.

Gonzales, R. A. NMDA receptors excite alcohol research. *Trends in Pharmacological Sciences* 11:137–139, 1990.

Nahas, G. *Marihuana: Chemistry, Biochemistry, and Cellular Effects.* New York: Springer Verlag, 1976.

Robins, L., and Helzer, J. Narcotic use in Southeast Asia and afterward. *Archives of General Psychiatry* 32:955–961, 1975.

3

There's No Free Lunch

Goals

People take drugs because these substances make them feel good and decrease some "bad" feelings. The first time a substance is tried, each person is convinced that the drug will be pure enough, the dose low enough, and the ability to control future use strong enough that few if any dangers are involved. Each person convinces him- or herself that drug use is "a free lunch" with no associated problems.

However, all of the drugs covered in this text have things in common. They are taken into the body relatively easily, quickly enter into the bloodstream, and have rapid effects on the brain. They *all* have a way of making us feel high or in some ways "better," and therefore all cause a level of psychological dependence. This means once regular use begins, they are likely to become objects of desire for you, and you would rather continue with the drug than stop using it.

This would not necessarily be a problem if it were not for the price you have to pay for continued use. Unfortunately, repeated intake of these substances causes a range of difficulties, including medical consequences, the possibility of physical addiction, as well as problems with brain functioning, including states of confusion, psychosis, and intense feelings of depression or anxiety.

This chapter discusses the price that often has to be paid for repeated heavy use of alcohol and other drugs of abuse. My philosophy is that you will more easily make a decision for yourself once you know the whole picture. Chapter 2 taught you about the types of drugs; this one reviews the patterns of problems associated with each drug category.

What Types of Problems Can Develop?

You learned in Chapter 2 about how drugs of abuse can be placed into categories based on their most usual effects at the usual doses. These groups are also helpful in understanding more about the pattern of problems likely to be seen with a particular type of drugs. All of the substances cause psychological dependence, all have some medical problems associated with them, and all can cause some form of temporary psychological problems. However, the likelihoods of developing confusion, psychosis (a state of craziness), depression, and anxiety are quite different for the different drug categories. Similarly, not all of these substances cause physical withdrawal symptoms when use is stopped.

The third section of this chapter tells you the pattern of problems most closely related to each group of drugs. However, before getting down to the specific dangers associated with different drugs, I want to give a more general description of what the problems can be.

Medical Problems

Taken in the amounts used to get high, none of the substances of abuse are really "natural" to your bodies the way vitamins or minerals might be. Therefore, each body organ has to find a way to cope with a "foreign" substance, with the liver, the kidneys, and the lungs carrying the added burden of eliminating the drug from the body. Whereas occasional exposure to most of these agents causes a kind of organ "bruising" from which the body almost always recovers, very high doses or repeated exposure can produce more long-lasting and sometimes permanent problems. These can include the potential sequelae discussed below.

An Overdose

An overdose usually means that so much of the alcohol or drug has reached the brain that the essential body activities can no longer be carried out properly. Problems can develop with breathing, keeping the blood pressure in the normal range, maintaining a regular heartbeat, or regulating body temperature. Sometimes, either the drug itself or the associated interference with normal brain functioning causes a surge of brain electrical activity that is expressed as a convulsion.

Although almost any drug is theoretically capable of causing a lethal overdose, this is especially likely with the depressants, the opiates, and the stimulants. Death can occur within a matter of minutes. Treatment involves helping the body to keep the breathing, blood pressure, and other functions going until the liver or kidneys or lungs can get rid of the drug and the brain can function normally once again. Rarely, machines can be used to help filter the substance out of the blood, a process called dialysis.

The Consequences of IV Drug Use

As you have seen in Chapter 1, there are serious dangers associated with administering drugs through unsterile needles and syringes. This practice can overwhelm the body with bacteria that can cause infections of some of the body organs (a **large abscess**) and can produce a condition that can destroy the heart valves (**bacterial endocarditis**). Drugs taken intravenously can also expose the body to other infectious material, the most dangerous and deadly of which is the acquired immune deficiency syndrome (AIDS) virus. This means, of course, that if intravenous (IV) users limited themselves to sterile needles and syringes, many of the life-threatening dangers could be avoided. Because of the severity of the problems seen for most IV users, it is worth taking a bit more time to review some further details of these severe medical consequences that can occur with IV use.

In humans, AIDS is caused by a virus that attacks the body's immune system, producing a lethal vulnerability to infections and to cancers. The body normally controls these dangers through immune functioning, but once the body has been infected with this virus, it can no longer always monitor and control pathological invaders. The virus often sits dormant in the body for months or years after the infection. At this stage, antibodies to the virus can be detected in the blood, and the person is considered positive for the HIV virus or "HIV positive." The earliest signs of an immune problem generally occur when there is a decrease in the number of some very important types of white blood cells known as T-cells. The condition, which is among the earliest stages of the AIDS syndrome, is often referred to as AIDS-related complex or ARC, as opposed to the full-blown AIDS condition with its associated infections and unusual cancers such as Kaposi's sarcoma. Subsequently, clinical infections such as a pneumonia or the unusual cancers appear, at which stage the person is considered to have the AIDS condition itself.

Two other severe medical complications of IV drug use are also worth mentioning. Bacterial endocarditis is a bacterial infection of the internal lining of the heart—tissue referred to as the **endocardium.** Therefore, endocarditis is the inflammation ("itis") of the heart lining. One vulnerable tissue in the inside of the heart makes up the valves that are present between the four chambers of the heart and that control the direction and efficiency of the flow of blood. The infections often result in destruction of part of the valve which, of course, impairs the heart's ability to pump blood, and produces a life-threatening condition.

The third major consequence of IV drug use that we briefly review here involves an infection ("itis") of the liver (referred to in medical jargon as the **hepatic organ**) known as hepatitis. This infection of the liver can occur from a variety of conditions. Alcoholics develop an inflammation of their liver related to the manner in which alcohol directly injures liver cells, whereas other people can develop hepatitis through eating food that has been contaminated with a virus that attacks the liver. However, a very potent liver-destroying virus is spread through tainted syringes and needles. Therefore, IV drug users who share syringes or needles have a great chance of spreading the blood-borne hepatitis virus to their drug-using associates. Unfortunately, because the body only has one liver, any overwhelming infection of this organ can be lethal.

Accidents

Any substance that decreases the level of alertness, impairs judgment, or increases the amount of time it takes for the body to react when something happens can have another deadly consequence by increasing the chance of an accident at work, at home, while driving, or while playing. Therefore, substances, especially the depressants, marijuana-type drugs, and opiates, play an important role in contributing to the second or third leading cause of death in the United States: auto accidents, falls, fires, and drowning.

Other Medical Problems

Some substances cause a deterioration of vital organs such as the heart, liver, kidney, and brain. Other drugs destroy the lungs, some produce a deterioration of the lining of the nose and throat, some decrease the body's ability to fight off infections, and others cause increases in the risk for cancer.

Physical Dependence or Addiction and the Withdrawal or Abstinence Syndrome

As many of you already know, repeated intake of any of the opiates, brain depressants, and stimulants causes compensatory changes in the body. The result is that when you stop using these drugs after taking them in high enough doses for a long enough period of time, you will experience withdrawal symptoms.

In general, what develops during withdrawal is the *opposite* of what the drug usually does the first several times it is used. Therefore, for example, withdrawal from stimulants includes feelings of depression, sleepiness, and lack of confidence; the abstinence syndrome for some depressants includes anxiety, insomnia, and increase in blood pressure and temperature; and withdrawal from opiates involves pain, diarrhea, and a cough. For drugs that originally produced relatively short-lasting highs, these symptoms are most severe for the first several days after abstinence or cutting back on use, and then improve over the next three or four days. For drugs that produce long-lasting highs such as methadone or Valium, the initial symptoms of withdrawal might not be seen for several days or a week after stopping, and they might persist for several weeks or so. In either event some more mild symptoms remain, however, and these can take an additional period of two to six months or so to disappear.

This longer term or **protracted abstinence syndrome** is worth a few words. Many health care providers and most substance-dependent people expect that once the acute withdrawal or abstinence syndrome is over, usually in less than a week, the person returns to normal. Unfortunately, even though the person who has been physically addicted to a drug is likely to be greatly improved by the end of that first week or so, bothersome symptoms remain for several months. These tend to be quite subtle and thus are sometimes ignored. One important symptom is a feeling of "unease" because the heart and breathing rates are not responding adequately to changes in the environment. Other common symptoms of protracted withdrawal syndrome, seen with depressants, stimulants, and opiates, are feelings of nervousness and problems sleeping. Because the symptoms are so subtle and because at least subconsciously most people recognize that the problems will temporarily improve if they go back to their drug of abuse, it is likely that the protracted abstinence syndrome adds significantly to the risk for relapse. Although there are no formal treatments for protracted withdrawal, knowing that these feelings are "normal," that they will disappear with continued abstinence, and that they do not mean something is inherently wrong with the individual can be very reassuring.

Confusion

Confusion occurs when people have trouble thinking things through and are unsure about where they are and what is going on around them. Becoming intoxicated with any brain depressant such as alcohol causes confusion, as does intoxication with any of the solvent inhalants such as gasoline or with phencyclidine (PCP). Going through physical withdrawal from brain depressant drugs such as alcohol or the Valium-type benzodiazepines can also cause severe temporary confusion. Although all of these conditions are likely to disappear within several days to several weeks (except for PCP, where the confusion can remain for several months), a few drugs can cause such severe brain damage that confusion never goes away. For example, this can happen after many years of heavy drinking of alcohol and after repeated intoxication with the solvent inhalants.

Psychosis (Craziness)

Drugs are probably the most common reason that people develop temporary symptoms of severe psychosis. Almost all people who take high enough doses of any of the stimulants will begin to think people are plotting against them (a **paranoid delusion**), and most will begin to hear voices they think are real (**auditory hallucinations**). A small proportion of men and women who are using brain depressants such as alcohol heavily will develop similar symptoms. Thankfully, these symptoms almost always disappear within several weeks to a month or so of abstinence.

Depression and Anxiety

As used here, the term **depression** indicates a condition where a person is sad and blue, has lost self-confidence, is having trouble sleeping or is sleeping all the time, feels like crying, feels guilty, and is likely to see the future as hopeless. When a condition like this goes on all day every day for weeks on end, it is called a major depression.

Symptoms that resemble these depressions are common with repeated intoxication with depressant drugs and are a central part of the withdrawal symptoms following physical addiction to the stimulants. These depressions can be so severe that the person thinks of suicide. A less intense depression can also occur with repeated intake of opiates, such as methadone, heroin, or some prescription painkillers.

The term **anxiety** indicates a level of nervousness that is intense enough and long-lasting enough to impair a person's normal level of functioning. The specific symptoms induced can vary greatly. For example, sometimes anxiety is seen as a high level of nervousness and worrying, sometimes it comes on as a ten- to thirty-minute period of a severe panic attack (where the heart beats fast and hard, and it is hard to catch your breath), and other times people become frightened of leaving the house or of mixing in with crowds. Temporary anxiety states like these are likely to be seen during stimulant intoxication, even when the stimulants are as weak as caffeine or diet pills. These symptoms can also occur during withdrawal from brain depressants like alcohol.

Anxiety or depressive states caused by substances tend to be intense during drug use and for perhaps several days to a month following stopping the drug. Some symptoms of nervousness may then linger off and on for a period of two to six months or so as a protracted abstinence syndrome, with the intensity of the problem improving with each passing week. It is unlikely that any drug causes permanent depression or permanent severe anxiety.

Other Problems

Substances that find their way to many different parts of the body and have strong effects on the brain can produce a host of other problems. One possible difficulty is a **flashback,** which means feeling high or intoxicated again after the drug effects have originally worn off. This usually is experienced as a wave of feeling that occurs days, and even weeks, after the last drug dose. This condition, almost always temporary, is most likely to be seen with the marijuana-type drugs and the hallucinogens.

A second condition is **violence.** People tend to strike out when they are extremely agitated, confused, and frustrated. Therefore, any drug that causes confusion, depression, agitation, or any combination of the three will increase the chance that violence will occur. This means that a violent condition can occur after taking any of the depressants, the stimulants, and PCP, and can also be seen with the hallucinogens, and even with the solvents.

Another problem is **danger to the fetus,** or baby growing inside the womb. Most drugs easily cross in the blood to the developing baby. Every substance that is discussed in this text affects the functioning of many different body organs, including the brain. Therefore, theoretically, any drug of abuse is dangerous for a pregnant woman and her developing baby. The most impressive amount of evidence regarding problems in the development of the fetus is seen with alcohol and tobacco. Alcohol increases the rate of spontaneous abortions, can produce mental retardation, heart problems, and an abnormally small size of the baby.

Which Drugs Have Which Types of Problems? (See Table 3.1)

The Stimulants

Medical Problems

Use of stimulants (such as amphetamines and cocaine) can lead to a host of severe medical problems. A life-threatening overdose causes extremely high body temperatures, such high blood pressure that a stroke can develop, such severe abnormalities of the heart beating pattern that the heart can stop, as well as possible violent convulsions. Other medical problems can occur as a result of the method one uses to take a stimulant, including the entire group of difficulties seen with any IV drug use, potential damage to the lungs from inhaling crack or freebase cocaine smoke, and ulcers of the lining of the nose and throat

Table 3.1
Likely Dangers[a] Associated with Major Drugs

Drug group	Medical	Lethal overdose	Physical addiction	Temporary confusion	Temporary psychosis	Temporary depression	Temporary anxiety
Stimulants	+	+	+	−	+	+	+
Depressants	+	+	+	+	+	+	+
Opiates	+	+	+	−	−	Mild	−
Marijuana	+	−	−	−	−	Mild	−
Hallucinogens	+	−	−	For PCP	−	Mild	Mild
Solvents and inhalants	+	−	−	+	−	−	−

[a]This list does *not* give all possible dangers. It only notes prominent problems likely to be seen with each drug.

from snorting these drugs. Other dangers include high blood pressure and heartbeat irregularities.

Physical Addiction and Withdrawal

All of the stimulants are physically addicting. Repeated use produces a need for higher doses to get an effect (tolerance), and actual physical addiction is likely to develop within a day or two of repeated use. The withdrawal syndrome begins within hours of the last dose and consists of severe depression, lack of energy, a great need for sleep, and a marked increase in appetite. These are most prominent for the first week of abstinence, and may persist at a decreasing level for several months. Some feelings of depression and mood swings can remain for as long as six months.

Psychosis

This group of drugs is the one most likely to cause a temporary psychosis that is characterized by hallucinations and/or thinking people are plotting to harm you. Here, after as few as two or three administrations over a period of several hours or even one large dose, people often begin to feel an early sign that a psychosis is developing, a belief that someone is watching or plotting against them. This can rapidly develop into a determined feeling by the user that he or she is in real danger of physical harm. These feelings are often accompanied by voices either inside or outside the head that either comment on what one is doing, or that call out names, or instruct the person to carry out certain actions. During this period of time, stimulant abusers are not confused in that they can otherwise think clearly and know where they are and what is going on around them. This severe psychotic state is sometimes misdiagnosed as schizophrenia, a serious, often life-long psychiatric condition. Stimulant-induced psychoses, however, are almost always temporary, and tend to improve within a matter of days and disappear within several days to weeks after the drug is stopped.

Depression and Anxiety

Depression is a consistent after-effect of any regular use of a stimulant. If use was long enough and the dose high enough to cause physical addiction, during the withdrawal syndrome the sadness can be so intense that people attempt suicide. The good news is that within several days to a week the depression is likely to improve greatly, with lingering symptoms decreasing gradually over the following months.

The use of any drug where intoxication increases the heart rate and blood pressure is also likely to produce severe **anxiety.** Taking high levels of any stimulant, even caffeine, can cause the heart to beat fast and hard, can cause intense nervousness, produce a trembling of the hands, and can create a feeling of dread and a fear of interacting with other people or moving about in crowds. Because these symptoms can be quite severe, these temporary problems can be misdiagnosed as an anxiety disorder. Thankfully, the anxiety is likely to improve and then disappear with time after use of the drug has stopped.

Other Problems

One of the most dangerous effects of repeated stimulant use is **violence.** The combination of feeling overstimulated and highly suspicious can cause users to strike out and even commit murder.

Finally, stimulants easily cross into the bloodstream and brain of the **developing fetus.** This does not appear to produce malformations but can cause severe physical addiction in the infant. After birth, a withdrawal syndrome including lethargy, irritability, and feeding problems can be seen in the baby. While this condition is likely to improve within weeks, some learning and behavioral problems can last much longer.

The Depressants

It's not by chance that I have discussed the dangers of the stimulants and depressants first. For all sorts of reasons, the stimulant drugs and the depressants have the most stark pattern of dangers associated with them.

Medical Problems

The medical problems seen during repeated use of the depressants can be truly frightening. Among members of this group of drugs (which also include barbiturates and the Valium-type drugs), alcohol is the most commonly used and probably disrupts the greatest diversity of body systems when taken in high doses on a regular basis.

Just touching on some of the most obvious consequences, there is a greatly increased risk for *infections* and perhaps a ten-times higher level of various types of *cancers* among alcoholics than is seen in the general population. Alcohol increases both blood pressure and the harmful types of blood fats. The result is an increased risk of *stroke* and *heart attack*. Alcohol in high doses can also affect the *liver*, causing a serious inflammation (**alcoholic hepatitis**) and cell destruction resulting in excessive scarring of the liver (**cirrhosis**). During bouts of heavy drinking, the *blood-producing systems* have difficulty making adequate blood products such as red and white blood cells. There is also an *impaired production* of the blood components responsible for appropriate clotting (the **platelets**). The *nerves* to the hands and feet can be slowly destroyed over many years of heavy drinking in a way that produces severe and often permanent "pins and needles" and numbness (**peripheral neuropathy**). The ability of men and women to produce the usual pattern of *sex hormones* is also likely to be impaired, so that men often develop problems with sexual functioning (**impotence**) and women experience menstrual irregularities.

The early stages of each of these problems is reversible. However, if heavy drinking continues, the damage can be permanent and at times life-threatening. The other brain depressants, including the Valium-type drugs and the barbiturates, cause some similar impairments, especially in the brain, but they do not produce the same wide pattern of destruction seen with alcohol.

The depressant drugs are also very dangerous in *overdose*. Indeed, probably the most common cause of deaths by overdose in the United States involves alcohol. Here, as would be true of an overdose of any depressant, high doses of alcohol produce a deep sleep, which is soon followed by a shutdown of the breathing and heartbeat regulating centers of the brain, with subsequent death.

These drugs can also greatly impair the ability to think quickly and react appropriately and, therefore, are probably the most common substances involved in *fatal accidents* on the road, at work, or in the home. Although most of the depressants are taken orally, some forms of barbiturates and the Valium-type drugs are taken IV. In this case, the use of nonsterile needles creates all of the risks of IV drugs.

Physical Addiction and Withdrawal

Physical addiction is a major potential problem with all depressants. The withdrawal syndrome that develops after taking increasing doses of any of these drugs can be severe. The average person undergoing withdrawal from alcohol, the Valium-type drugs, or the barbiturates has a mild-to-moderate syndrome that involves trouble sleeping, anxiety, a tremor of the hands, and increases in the pulse rate, blood pressure, breathing rate, and body temperature. During withdrawal, a small proportion of users experience convulsions or severe states of confusion. All of these withdrawal states are likely to be most intense over the first several days after stopping use of the drug. They then markedly decrease by day four or five, and then continue to slowly improve over the next several months. An exception to this time frame occurs for the drugs that stay in the body for long periods of time (such as Valium and Librium [chlordiazepoxide]), where symptoms might not begin until a week or so after stopping the drug and could remain with high intensity for several weeks to a month.

Confusion

Getting high from any of the depressants usually involves problems with thinking, impaired balance, a loss of clarity of speech, and problems with coordination. Sometimes the effect is so intense that the user appears confused and may have trouble caring for himself or herself. Some people, especially older individuals and others with brain damage, are likely to become confused after even low doses of depressants (including two or three drinks or what would be considered usual prescribed doses of the Valium-type drugs). Unfortunately, this temporary confusion caused by depressants could be misdiagnosed as some sort of brain deterioration such as Alzheimer's disease. The confusion caused by depressants is likely to improve over a period of days to weeks, but, if it is misdiagnosed as Alzheimer's, people might be given inappropriate treatments.

Psychosis

Although not occurring as commonly as with the stimulants where almost anyone will develop hallucinations or delusions if the dose of the drug is high enough, severe states of a temporary psychosis can also result in some people from use of depressants. A short-lived psychosis has been associated most clearly with alcohol, but there are hints that the barbiturates and the Valium-type drugs can bring on temporary psychotic symptoms where the user believes people are plotting against him or her and hears voices. These conditions often develop rapidly without any warning, even in men and women who have been using the depressants for a high off and on for many years. If this type of psychosis does occur, it looks just like a major psychiatric disorder (schizo-phrenia), and can be misdiagnosed by psychiatrists and psychologists. Although the symptoms of psychosis can be frightening, with complete abstinence the voices and severe paranoid thoughts are likely to fade away within days to weeks.

Anxiety and Depression

The depressant drugs are aptly named because these are probably the most common drugs of abuse that cause severe *depression* of mood during intoxication. Several studies have shown that anyone who takes high doses of a depressant drug such as alcohol is likely to show feelings of being irritated, have problems sleeping, develop difficulties concentrating, and have feelings of sadness. The higher the dose of the depressants and the longer the period of time they are taken, the more intense the depression will be. It should not be surprising, therefore, that after drinking heavily for many days, one-half to two-thirds of alcoholics have some severe signs of depression. Similarly, it is an unfortunate but well-documented statistic that at least 10% of alcoholics commit suicide during such depressions (1). This is terribly sad because if the alcoholic can sober up and remain abstinent, the depression is almost certain to improve markedly in a matter of days to weeks and then totally disappear over a period of several weeks to months of abstinence.

Similarly, withdrawal from brain depressant drugs has a very high rate of associated symptoms of *anxiety*. In one study, 80% of alcoholics going through withdrawal complained of episodes of trouble catching their breath and of palpitations (with the heart beating fast and hard) of such severity that it looked like a panic attack (2). Also, probably one-third or more of alcoholics (and those who have had problems with other brain depressants) have such high levels of anxiety in the weeks during acute and pro-tracted withdrawal that they have problems making themselves go out of the house, have great difficulty feeling comfortable with crowds, and complain of discomfort at parties or situations where they have to mix with other people. Fortunately, these symptoms that resemble the anxiety conditions called social phobia and agoraphobia are also likely to improve rapidly over the subsequent weeks and then totally disappear.

Other Problems

Women who drink alcohol while pregnant run the risk of causing severe damage to the unborn children. This occurs because alcohol and the products the body makes when breaking down this chemical are easily transported to the developing baby in the womb. Whereas the danger of fetal damage increases with higher amounts and frequencies of alcohol consumption, there is no known safe level of alcohol consumption during pregnancy. This is why most doctors and the United States Surgeon General recommend that women completely abstain from alcohol for the full nine months of pregnancy. Just as alcohol can severely damage the health of the adult drinker, it can cause devastating problems for the unborn child. These problems can include mental retardation, heart defects, abnormalities in the shape of the nose and eyelids, low birth weight with continued stunted growth throughout life, and a variety of other difficulties. This group of symptoms is known as the fetal alcohol syndrome (FAS). Unfortunately for the alcohol-damaged child and his or her family, FAS is irreversible.

Finally, the brain depressants, especially alcohol, are closely associated with many forms of *violence*. This is probably a result of the irritability, tiredness, and feelings of loss of control that these drugs can cause.

The Opiates

Heroin, codeine, almost all of the prescription painkillers, and all of the rest of the drugs described under this heading in Chapter 2 have a predictable pattern of problems. These result from the manner in which these drugs are taken into the body (IV) and the rapidity with which physical addiction can develop to these substances.

Medical Problems

People who use opiates IV (most usually heroin) run the entire range of problems described in Chapter 2 for the IV route. Many opiate users turn to IV administration because of the rapid, intense, and clear high that is produced. Once experienced, this is a pattern of intake that is very difficult to give up. In addition, the opiates are lethal in overdose, usually producing a rapid shutdown in breathing and heartbeat. They also sometimes cause death by producing changes that fill the lungs with fluid and impair the ability of the body to get adequate levels of oxygen.

Physical Addiction

This condition can develop very quickly when any of the opiates are used repeatedly for a high. For the drugs that only remain in the body for several hours, such as heroin, withdrawal symptoms are likely to be experienced every four hours or so. This means that the user needs to take the drug regularly, and that every morning he or she is greeted with withdrawal symptoms upon awakening. These symptoms include a feeling of pain everywhere in the body (especially muscles and joints), nervousness, inability to sleep well, stomach pains associated with nausea, vomiting, diarrhea, "goose bumps" and a painful feeling of the skin, problems controlling the body's temperature, along with a runny nose and cough. For almost all of the substances, except methadone (a drug that lingers in the body for many hours), withdrawal symptoms are likely to be at their maximum one to two days after stopping the drug and then markedly decrease by day four or five of abstinence. However, some feelings of unease and levels of mood swings continue for several months. Because methadone remains in the body for a long time, symptoms of withdrawal from this drug don't begin until a week or so after stopping use, and they probably remain moderately intense for three to four weeks.

Thus, other than the severe consequences associated with IV administration, the major problems associated with opiates are medical (including overdoses) and the consequences of physical addiction. States of confusion are unlikely during intoxication or withdrawal, and problems with depression tend to be relatively mild, with symptoms of nervousness or anxiety most likely to be associated with a craving for the drug when it is not available. Most other types of complications are not prominent here.

The Marijuana-type Drugs

With the exception of alcohol and caffeine, these drugs (especially marijuana tobacco and hashish) are more widely used in most Western countries than any other drug discussed in this text. It is likely that in some settings more people in the United States smoke marijuana than use tobacco products (3). Despite this widespread use and a general belief that the drugs might not be very dangerous, the cannabinols have a substantial number of problems associated with their use.

Medical Problems

Most of the difficulties associated with marijuana fall under this heading. Even though this group of drugs is virtually never taken IV and rarely (if ever) causes a fatal overdose, regular use is associated with a host of potentially severe consequences. By far the most obvious of these problems is the way that marijuana-type drugs impair the judgment, coordination, and reaction time essential for safe *driving*. Because the drug remains in the body for such a long time, this impairment in driving ability is likely to be observed for more than eight hours after smoking a marijuana cigarette. Complicating the picture even more is the manner in which the active ingredient in marijuana, THC, becomes dissolved in fat stores in the body, and is subsequently released in a manner that can cause a level of impairment the following day or even the day after that. It is probable that, with the exception of alcohol, the marijuana-type drugs contribute to more accident deaths in the United States than any other substance. This is not only because of the effects the drug has, but because, even more than with alcohol, people seem to have little understanding of how impaired they are. So, they might be more likely to drive when high on the drug than they would be if high on alcohol.

Other medical problems are equally serious, although they take longer to develop. Marijuana smoke is extremely irritating and full of tars. Thus, it produces an *irritation of the lungs* and air tubes (bronchitis), while also increasing symptoms of asthma. The smoke has four-to-ten times higher levels of cancer-producing agents than tobacco smoke, and probably increases the risk for mouth, throat, and lung cancer among heavy smokers. Additional medical problems seen with regular use of these drugs include mild levels of impairment in the body's immune system, and a reduction in the body's ability to produce adequate levels of some hormones, including those that affect sexual development.

Psychoses

It is not likely that these drugs directly cause people to hear voices (except when high) or become very suspicious. However, at least one convincing long-term study has indicated that regular use does increase the chances that people who are at high risk for psychiatric disorders such as schizophrenia will develop their disorder earlier in their lives.

Other Problems

There are a number of remaining problems. These include *flashbacks*, or feelings of becoming high again hours or days after the last intake of marijuana. This can be frightening, interferes with school, work, and driving performance, and is often a cause of increased levels of *anxiety*. An additional difficulty is that the lingering levels of the drug tend to cause a *lack of energy and motivation* that can make it difficult to accomplish tasks for days after the drug is stopped. For a person who consumes this drug multiple times a week, the lack of focus and motivation is likely to be present all the time. Thankfully, the problem is likely to disappear within several weeks or a month of abstinence.

Hallucinogens

Even though this group contains a variety of types of drugs, it's still possible to present some general conclusions regarding the types of problems likely to be encountered with their use.

Medical Problems

Although most of the hallucinogens (LSD, mescaline, and peyote) are not closely associated with obvious medical problems, one potential danger is that repeated heavy use of these drugs might interfere with normal brain functioning, thus temporarily impairing the user's ability to think things through clearly. Another potential medical problem has been reported with the hallucinogen methylene dioxyamphetamine (MDA) and its relative, 3,4-methylenedioxymethamphetamine (MDMA or Ecstasy) (4). These drugs are likely to attack areas of the brain rich in a specific chemical (serotonin), with the development of subsequent neurological problems. Various forms of the hallucinogen STP might cause severe impairment of the circulation of blood to the arms and legs. On the other hand, overdose deaths are rarely reported with the hallucinogens, and, considering how rapidly they are distributed in the body by other avenues of administration, there is no reason to take the drugs IV.

Psychosis

It might seem surprising that the hallucinogens are not likely to cause a condition of severe psychosis. Indeed, the "high" from these drugs rarely involves actual hallucinations, but more often centers on feelings of an increased depth of the ability to hear, see, and experience the environment. Even when hallucinations do occur, they are likely to involve seeing geometric shapes of various colors and lights. Thus, the users, while frightened, are not likely to appear to be crazy because they realize that the drug has caused the high (that is, they have insight).

Depression and Anxiety

Similarly, although the hallucinogens cause feelings of anxiety and can increase feelings of depression, this is temporary and only likely to be seen during or soon after intoxication. Of course, anxiety is not unexpected because many of the hallucinogens have stimulating properties, and some are even closely related to the amphetamines. Levels of depression associated with the hallucinogens can be intense, but are usually short-lived, often disappearing as the intoxication goes away.

Confusion

Intoxication with PCP is likely to produce severe agitation along with confusion—a combination that is likely to result in violence and physical injury. The decreased ability to think brought on by this drug is very frightening to those around the user, especially because, unlike states of confusion seen with most drugs, a PCP-induced confused state can remain for two or three months.

Other Problems

Flashbacks are probably observed with the hallucinogens more than with any other drug. The most frequent experience is seeing lights, colors, or shapes, especially when going from a bright place to a darker environment. These episodes, usually lasting only a matter of minutes, can be very frightening and the visions can interfere with one's ability to drive at night. However, the experiences are only temporary and are likely to stop oc-curring within days to weeks.

Another area of great concern with the hallucinogens is the possibility that they might cause changes in the strands of genes in the cells called chromosomes, and subsequently produce *fetal damage.* This is a real concern, although it is impossible to prove because most people who take hallucinogens are also using a variety of other substances. Nonetheless, hallucinogens are potent drugs, they may create a danger in the normal development of the fetus, and there are some indications that they might produce an increased rate of spontaneous abortions and fetal abnormalities in the offspring of users.

The Solvents and Inhalants

The two major problems (in addition to psychological dependence) associated with these drugs involve medical conditions and confusion.

Medical Problems

These difficulties are prominent with inhalants because of their ability to rapidly interfere with functioning of the heart, liver, kidneys, lungs, and brain. Heartbeat irregularities (called **arrhythmias**) often occur during use of any of these substances and can sometimes be fatal. The *liver* carries the major brunt of attempts of the body to rid itself of the solvents, and these sub-stances are toxic enough that an inflammation of the liver can easily develop (**hepatitis**). This is usually reversible but can some-times be associated with permanent damage.

Many inhalants and solvents are also excreted from the body by the *kidneys,* and at least two solvents (toluene and benzene), substances that are found in most inhalants used to cause a high, can cause permanent kidney damage. The *lungs* are the doorway through which these substances enter the bloodstream, and when taken in higher concentration, the solvents almost always temporarily interfere with the ability of the lungs to gather enough oxygen. Additional difficulties include temporary destruction of body muscle as the solvents are carried in the bloodstream throughout the body, decreases in the production of all types of blood cells that can result in a life-threatening type of anemia, and a solvent-produced destruction of the nerves to the hands and feet, similar to the effects of alcohol (a peripheral neuropathy).

The signs of intoxication with solvents certainly indicate that the brain does not tolerate these substances very well. Most people have difficulty thinking, a lightheadedness, and complain of headaches during and immediately following a "high." These symptoms are usually accompanied by alterations in the usual brain wave pattern. There is a great deal of evidence that long-term repeated intake of solvents can result in a permanent brain damage, where the user develops a tremor of the hands, an unsteady walking gait, a weak voice, and permanent difficulty with thinking clearly.

Confusion

One of the most common difficulties associated with the use of solvents or inhalants is the intoxication-related confusion, thinking impairment, and inability to carry out even relatively simple tasks that can be very disturbing not only to users but to those around them.

Depression and Anxiety

Temporary psychological problems can include mild levels of anxiety and depression, but these are not usually prominent.

Other Drugs

 This section briefly describes difficulties associated with some other drugs of potential abuse. These drugs all cause psychological dependence, all are capable of producing temporary periods of anxiety and depression (although these are not as severe as those observed with the depressants and the stimulants), but none are physically addicting. The major difficulties are likely to involve medical problems or states of confusion.

Amyl and Butyl Nitrite ("Poppers")

"Poppers" are not only of concern because of the *confusion* they can cause during intoxication and their ability to produce *psychological dependence,* but they can produce a potentially serious *drop in blood pressure.* These drugs can also cause people to have severe attacks of *panic,* interfere with the ability of the blood to carry *oxygen* to the body organs, and probably *impair the body's ability to fight off infections and cancers.*

Nitrous Oxide (Laughing Gas)

This substance can produce a temporary *psychosis* that disappears very rapidly, causes poor judgment and incoordination with a resulting heightened risk for *accidents,* and is thought to possibly interfere with the body's *immune functions.*

Over-the-Counter (OTC) Drugs

Some nonprescription agents can also be abused and cause a variety of difficulties. The *antihistamines,* used in over-the-counter sleeping pills and tranquilizers, can produce confusion and enough fatigue to interfere with driving skills; overuse of many of the *decongestant* cold or hay fever drugs can markedly raise the blood pressure and cause severe mood swings; repeated heavy daily use of most over-the-counter *pain pills* (containing phenacetin, acetaminophen, and ibuprophin) can destroy both the kidneys and liver; while over-the-counter *stimulants* like No-Doz and Vivarin (containing 100 to 200 milligrams of caffeine) increase the blood pressure and are likely to cause both temporary anxiety and depression.

Anabolic Steroids

Overuse of other types of prescription pills can also cause severe problems. Probably the most common additional prescription drugs that don't fall into any of the categories discussed thus far are the *anabolic steroids* used by muscle builders. These substances are similar in structure to the male hormone, testosterone, and help the body to retain some important muscle building blocks like nitrogen. However, when used on a regular basis, the anabolic steroids cause *mood swings*, possibly contribute to acts of *violence*, and occasionally cause psychoses. They also produce a variety of severe *medical problems*, including liver cancers and stunted bone growth (with a subsequent short stature if begun in early adolescence), cause women to develop male-pattern sex characteristics, produce impotence in men, and so on.

A Note to Family and Friends

This chapter is actually written as much for your use as for reading by someone who is concerned about his or her own problem. My goal here has been to present as much information as possible about what drugs are and what problems they are likely to cause. To be of any use to you, it is important that the information be presented in a straightforward way. I have done everything I can to use the best data and to avoid anything that might sound like "scare tactics."

You can use the information given in this chapter in a way that will be most helpful to your family member or friend. This is actually part of the art of "intervention" that is discussed further in Chapter 6. The goal is to pick a time when the person you are concerned about is not intoxicated and when you are not in the middle of an argument with him or her. Thus, in a relaxed situation, the topic of your concern about substance use can be discussed, and you might share some of the information given here. It is important to help the person understand that the physical and emotional pain and discomfort they are going through was likely to be either caused by substances, or at least made worse by them. It is also important to point out how continued substance use is likely to cause an escalation of even more problems in the future. You might explain how damage might be done to specific organs by the particular type of substance, how continued use might lead to a temporary but severe state of craziness or psychosis, and discuss the potential for an overdose with lethal consequences.

Remember that intervention is never completed in "one shot." The process often requires continued concern and sharing of information in the hope that one of these times the person will be ready to "hear" what it is you have to say. Some people might actually prefer to read the information themselves. Perhaps asking them to review this chapter and the one before might be of use.

This is actually the first chapter in this text where I have deliberately set forth a section directed at family members and friends. This will become a regular part of each of the chapters in Part II.

A Recap

One important foundation of this text is that people need the best information possible when they are trying to make decisions. Therefore, where Chapter 2 described how the hundreds of substances people use for a "high" can be divided into a limited number of categories, this chapter takes the information one step further. The problems associated with substance use are relatively straightforward and fall into fairly obvious categories. These include the risk for psychological dependence (a property shared by all substances of abuse), potential medical difficulties, physical addiction (which is mostly a characteristic of the three classes of drugs including the depressants, stimulants, and opiates), severe confusion, psychosis (usually characterized by hearing voices and believing people are plotting against you), severe mood swings including depression and anxiety, and a variety of other problems including violence, flashbacks, and potential damage to the baby developing in the womb. There is a relatively unique pattern of these problems associated with each category of drug of abuse.

In putting this chapter together I have tried to pay most attention to the best studies that are available. Just as I feel that it is important for you to know which dangers are seen with which types of drugs, I have tried to be as honest as possible in helping you to recognize those dangers that are absent. You need the best information if you are going to make any of the important decisions that are now facing you.

Armed with the knowledge presented in Part I, you now have a feeling for what drugs are, what the intoxication is, and the pattern of dangers associated with substances. This knowledge is the first step in trying to decide whether you have a problem and what might be done about it.

Part I paves the way for the information offered in the following chapters that make up Part II. These are set up to allow you to consider whether there is really a problem, what factors might have contributed to the situation in which you might find yourself, and how you can begin to take the steps necessary to fight your way out of the difficulties. The chapters in Part II also offer some suggestions on how to find the more formal treatment program most appropriate for your own needs, and give an overview of what most programs try to do both during the active phase of treatment and in aftercare.

References

1. Murphy, G., Wetzel, R., Robins, E., and McEvoy, L. Multiple risk factors predict suicide in alcoholism. *Archives of General Psychiatry* 49:459–463, 1992.

2. Schuckit, M. A. Genetic and clinical implications of alcoholism and affective disorder. *American Journal of Psychiatry* 143:140–147, 1986.
3. Schuckit, M., Klein, J. L., Twitchell, G. R., and Springer, L. M. Increases in alcohol-related problems on a college campus. *J. Stud. Alc.* 55:739–742, 1994.
4. Battaglia, G., Yeh, S. Y., and DeSouza, E. B. MDMA-induced neurotoxicity. *Pharmacology Biochemistry and Behavior* 29:269–274, 1988.

Additional Readings

Beck, A., Steer, R., and Trexler, L. Alcohol abuse and eventual suicide. *Journal of Studies on Alcohol* 50:202–209, 1989.

Day, N. The effects of prenatal exposure to alcohol. *Alcohol Health and Research World* 16:238–244, 1992.

Dorus, M. *The Broken Cord*. New York: Harper & Row, 1989.

Metzger, D., Woody, G., De Philippis, D., McLellan, A., O'Brien, C., and Platt, J. Risk factors for needle sharing among methadone-treated patients. *American Journal of Psychiatry* 148:636–640, 1991.

Nwanyanwu, O., Chu, S., Green, T., Buehler, J., and Berkelman, R. Acquired immunodeficiency syndrome in the United States associated with injecting drug use, 1981–1991. *American Journal of Drug and Alcohol Abuse* 19:399–408, 1993.

Pohorecky, L., and Roberts, P. Development of tolerance to and physical dependence on ethanol: Daily versus repeated cycles treatment with ethanol. *Alcoholism: Clinical and Experimental Research* 15:824–833, 1991.

Silverman, K., Evans, S., Strain, E., and Griffiths, R. Withdrawal syndrome after the double-blind cessation of caffeine consumption. *New England Journal of Medicine* 327:1109–1113, 1992.

Stratton, K., Howe, C., and Battaglia, F. (eds.). *Fetal Alcohol Syndrome*. Washington, DC: National Academy Press, 1996.

Vaillant, G. *The Natural History of Alcoholism Revisited*. Cambridge, MA: Harvard University Press, 1995.

information, it would be appropriate to spend some time looking through the *Appendix* material related to Chapter 2. These cover:

1. *Suicidal Behavior and Substance Abuse.*
2. *Alcohol and Driving.*
3. *Are There Dangers to Marijuana?*
4. *Weight Lifter's Folly: The Abuse of Anabolic Steroids.*

Preface to Part II

The fact that you have turned to this page indicates that you have probably already either read (or at least browsed through) Part I. Or, perhaps you skipped the first section because you feel that more information relating to the nature of drugs is not your highest priority right now. In any event, there are probably a number of important questions that you are thinking about. So, I've organized my own thoughts around the types of information that you might need for yourself or for helping people around you when substance problems are involved.

Each chapter in Part II addresses a series of questions organized around a central theme. Chapter 4 focuses on some of the information you are likely to need if you are deciding whether you have a substance-related problem, whereas Chapter 5 deals with issues you might wrestle with if you are trying to figure out how you developed problems in the first place. Once a situation has developed, there are many questions you might ask about how you might start to *do* something to change the situation (Chapter 6), and other questions about how you might find the "right" program. (The quotation marks are there because, as discussed in Chapter 7, there are a variety of types of programs that are likely to work—not just one magical approach.) Next, if you decide where to go for help, you will want to know the type of information offered in Chapters 8 and 9, describing what is likely to happen during treatment. Then, all of the blood, sweat, and tears expended in winding your way through to that point in recovery combine to pave the way for Chapter 10, which talks about what still needs to be done after the formal treatment program has ended. I use Chapter 11 to pull together most of the major points that were offered to family and friends at different places in the text. The final chapter of the text pulls out all the information together in one summary.

Writing the series of chapters in Part II created some dilemmas for me. Part I is relatively straightforward because it is based solidly on good scientific data. In Part II, however, the scientific literature is less straightforward and not so easy to interpret. So, although I still use data, I have had to rely more on my personal and clinical experiences, and include a dose of my own opinions. Therefore, the information offered in this part of the book is a bit more controversial, and you may choose to supplement this information with some additional information and opinions.

A second issue relates to the fact that there are at least two types of readers for this book. There are those of you who are seeking information about whether you might have a problem and what to do about it. However, there are others who need guidance on how to help family members or friends who might have a substance problem. I have chosen to frame many of the questions as if the reader is asking about himself or herself—hopefully the second category of reader will have little problem translating a "you" to a "he" or "she." The exceptions are the sections within each chapter addressed directly to family and friends as well as Chapter 11. (By the way, I try to keep all comments applicable to men and women, but sometimes, just to keep the thoughts less "wordy," I use only "he" rather than "he and she.")

As a final comment before you plunge into the remaining work, I've tried to make the information as readable as possible by following the same basic flow of topics established in Part I. Each chapter begins with an introduction that sets out what it is I hope to accomplish, incorporates a section aimed specifically at families and friends of men and women with substance problems, and each ends with a Recap that reviews the major points I hope to have made. I also continue my practice of trying to give a quick answer to a question, which is then followed by some more complete thoughts to help those of you who want the maximum amount of information to best make up your mind on these "heady" issues. Of course, to give you access to more information, referrals to *Additional Readings* are offered.

I have spent enough time telling you what it is I am trying to do. Read on; I hope I'm able to offer some help.

4

Is There Really a Problem?

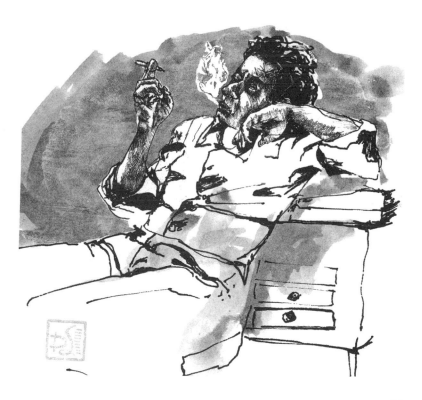

Figure 4.1. In this illustration, an individual is trying to make a decision. Similar to the situation in which many of you might find yourselves, he has already gathered enough knowledge to realize that drugs (ranging from nicotine to heroin) each pose dangers. On the other hand, giving up substance use will require changes in attitudes and lifestyles, consequences of abstinence that are not always easy to accept. This chapter outlines information that can be useful in attempting to decide whether or not a significant problem with substances exists.

Goals

By this point you have learned a bit about what drugs are, what they can do to you, and some risks you encounter when you take them. Now, you are facing a decision. Are the experiences that you have had with drugs or alcohol "normal," or is there a reason to seek help? I hope this chapter will help you to make up your mind.

You Can't Ask the Right Questions Unless You Get Rid of Inappropriate Stereotypes

Most of us have learned about alcohol, drugs, and the problems they cause through stories in movies, television, and popular magazines. Although the accuracy of these sources has improved in recent years, much of what the media have taught us has been reassuring but often wrong. It is comforting to think that the average drug abuser or alcoholic is easy to spot and is so different from us that we could never suffer a similar problem. At the same time, however, these visions blind us to the problems that we ourselves might be facing. This section presents a series of myths and the relevant facts that are often hidden by our attachment to inappropriate stereotypes of drug abusers and alcoholics.

Myth 1: The Average Alcoholic and Drug Abuser Lives on the Streets

Fifteen percent or more of the people in the United States and most other Western countries develop severe problems from alcohol, with at least 5% to 10% of people developing difficulties with other drugs (1). Even if you focus on the most severe and pervasive problems, at least 5% to 10% of the general population would actually meet medical criteria for alcohol dependence, with at least half again as many having diagnosable dependence on one type of drug or another. These figures represent very large numbers of people, the vast majority of whom never even see skid row, let alone live there. Most alcoholics and drug abusers have jobs and close relationships, they rarely (if ever) develop severe problems with the law, and many of them even go unrecognized as alcoholics or drug abusers by their physicians. Although most areas of these people's lives will eventually be impaired by their substance use, it is amazing how resilient people are and how they can continue to function (although at a relatively impaired level) for many years despite repeated substance use. Therefore, the average person with an alcohol or drug problem looks like the average person in society. She or he is likely to have a job or be in school, to have a family, and to appear to be relatively functional despite the drug problem. Many are professionals, artists, and community leaders.

Myth 2: People with Substance Problems Stay Intoxicated All the Time

Most people use their substances of choice more heavily on weekends, often abstaining on school and work days. Even during the days on which alcohol or drugs are taken, most users begin their day substance-free. Thus, the alcoholic or drug abuser is not constantly driven to take the drug. Rather, he or she is unable to limit use of the substance on a regular and predictable basis.

Myth 3: People with Substance Problems Have Terrible Problems Quitting

Even laboratory animals who have become physically addicted to heroin or alcohol through a research experiment and who have free access to the drug are likely to occasionally stop intake of the substance. It is almost as if they need to take a rest from the drug. Therefore, it should not be surprising that substance abusers regularly (sometimes almost weekly) test themselves by saying that they can stop—and they do. Since many people with alcohol and drug problems can achieve abstinence fairly easily, they use their ability to clean up or dry out to convince themselves that they do not have a problem with the substance and thus begin using again. After a period of use, the person again tests himself or herself by stopping intake of the drug. The ability to quit again convinces the individual that he or she does not have a problem, use is resumed, and the cycle of problems starts all over again. The key issue in a definition of an alcoholic- or drug-dependent person is that repeated problems eventually develop when the substances are used. Almost all of the people with these problems can and regularly do stop use temporarily.

Myth 4: People with Severe Substance Problems, Especially Those Having Difficulties Related to Alcohol, Never Control Their Substance Use

In the context of alcohol and drug dependence, rule-making becomes a common practice: you promise yourself that no alcohol will be consumed before 5:00 P.M., you will drink only beer (forgetting that 12 ounces of beer has about the same amount of alcohol as 1.0 to 1.5 ounces of bourbon and 4 ounces of wine), that you will only drink on weekends, or that you will never take alcohol in a special setting (like a party where relatives or the boss will be present). These rules, often established after a period of abstention where you have "proven" that stopping was not a problem, are often observed for days to months at a time. Such control is quite common! The problem is that once relatively severe substance-related problems have developed, it is *extremely uncommon* for the user to be able to maintain his or her control over substance intake for any extended period of time.

Soon after they have been established, the boundaries of the rules start to blur and fade as you begin to ask: if starting use at 5:00 P.M. is okay, what's wrong with starting at 4:00 P.M.? If I can limit myself to two drinks, what's wrong with three or four now and then? How could a small nightcap during the week hurt? Soon the borders around control disintegrate, the frequency and quantity of use escalate, and problems expand. The essential point is that once substance use begins, control is only temporary, and it is only a matter of time before new problems develop. The only way to guarantee no problems in the future for people with substance-related difficulties in the past is to stop using the drug altogether.

Myth 5: Most People with Severe Drug Problems Use Drugs IV

When we think of the drug-dependent person with "real" problems, most people tend to picture the opiate abuser who uses drugs IV. Unfortunately, because of this stereotype and the fact that IV drug use is exceptionally dangerous, we tend to downplay the dangers associated with the other drugs of choice. For example, marijuana is never taken IV, and yet severe levels of life impairment can occur from this drug. Most stimulant abusers (including those taking any of the various forms of cocaine or amphetamine) usually smoke or snort their drug and often pride themselves (while their lives are going down the tube) that they don't touch needles. Your common sense and your observations of the damage likely to be caused by alcohol certainly tell you that lives can (and are) easily destroyed by substances in the absence of any needles.

Myth 6: People with Substance Abuse Problems Can't Have Decent Moral Standards

It might make you feel safe to view alcoholics and drug abusers as having brought their problems on themselves because of low ethical standards and a lack of moral fortitude. However, many highly productive and ethical people have found themselves unable to control alcohol or other substance intake. These include responsible and admirable individuals such as Betty Ford, Elizabeth Taylor, Winston Churchill, and countless others.

In summary, if you want to find out whether you or those around you have a problem with substances, the first step is to drop your stereotypes. They make you feel safe, but the ignorance they produce might kill you.

Making a Good Decision Requires Knowing as Much as Possible about What Substance Use Problems are Like

By this point in your reading you know a great deal about what alcoholism and drug abuse and dependence are like, and you are aware of many of the erroneous stereotypes that can make deciding whether you have an alcohol or drug problem difficult. However, much of the information you have gained is likely to have come as a type of patchwork quilt, and it might be difficult to piece the whole picture together. Therefore, it is worth a few moments to talk about what substance problems are like for the mythical "average" person.

Beginning is Easy

Everyone begins drinking or taking drugs believing that use will be casual and problems will NEVER (I mean, NEVER) develop. Unfortunately, because of the nature of the "beast," minor problems soon start to occur, such as arguments that were never meant to happen, times you drove or participated in other risky behaviors while intoxicated, or times when you should have been at work or school but "partied" instead. At this early stage, things don't look a lot different for the developing alcoholic or drug-dependent person than they do for the general population.

However, continuing or returning to substance use *despite* these problems makes for far more frequent and more serious crises. This could be an alcoholic blackout when you can't remember how you got home from a party, or might include objections from your friends or spouse that alcohol or drugs are interfering with your relationships or costing too much money. Of course, it could be a more serious difficulty such as an automobile accident, a significant drop in grades, or an actual breakup of a relationship. The hard part is that these problems do not occur every day. One event develops one month and another might not appear until a few months later. However, if you look objectively, the pattern is there.

Denial of the Problems Then Develops

Substance abusers react to these crises in a variety of ways. Some people try to convince themselves that alcohol or drugs are not a problem by proving that they can stop using and/or control their substance intake for a period of time. Others convince themselves either that no problem exists, or that, although there might have been a substance-related accident or an interpersonal problem, the drugs or alcohol couldn't possibly be to blame. In either case, the pattern continues: substance use is eventually resumed, control is exerted for a limited period of time, but inevitably another problem pops up.

Here we get at the crux of whether an important alcohol or drug problem exists. All of the definitions described in Part I of this book boil down to one thing: **Continuing to take alcohol or drugs when they are causing life problems indicates that substance use has become more important to the user than the difficulties it causes.** Once this stage is reached, it is easy to predict that more problems are almost certain to develop once substance use resumes. These difficulties might not occur immediately, but as alcohol or drug intake becomes more regular and/or higher levels are taken, you can bet that more problems are just around the corner. The problems can include serious arguments with loved ones and friends while intoxicated or hungover, seriously impaired job or school performance, alcohol- and drug-related accidents, and evidence of damage to the brain, liver, heart, and so on.

When trying to decide whether you have a problem with drugs or alcohol, it is very important to make a distinction between occasional use (never a good thing, but not necessarily something that needs treatment) and regular use that results in problems. For example, studies show that somewhere between 40% and 70% of adolescents have tried marijuana at least once by the end of high school (2). On the other hand, only a small proportion of youth (probably less than 10%) use the marijuana-type drugs regularly—for example, three to seven times a week. Thus, although the majority of teenagers are likely to experiment with marijuana, a smaller number will develop a much more intense relationship with this drug. If the person then experiences life problems as a consequence of the drug use (such as difficulties at school, accidents, deteriorating relationships with relatives or peers, or brushes with the law) and still continues to take the drug, it is very probable that the problems will continue and escalate if this drug use continues.

Substance Problems Escalate

Now the plot thickens as the substance use takes on a life of its own. At this point, alcoholics or drug abusers begin to invest more time and more emotional energy in substance intake—they certainly demonstrate this by their willingness to continue to expose themselves to risk. Soon, the "beast" starts to awaken as events begin that solidify and even accelerate use of the substance.

For the user at this stage, friends who are light drinkers and who are not so involved with drugs usually start to drop away, leaving a peer group that not only doesn't discourage intake but actually urges more substance use. Problems are likely to develop within the "old" relationships, and these lead to fights (usually verbal, but sometimes physical). Unspoken rules get set up about what can and what cannot be talked about without precipitating an argument. The user develops an elaborate set of rationalizations to explain how the family does not understand, the boss is too demanding, and the laws don't make any sense. Each of these steps requires a greater level of psychological investment in continued use of alcohol or drugs. The higher the price you pay, the more important a substance becomes. Each consequence ups the ante yet another notch.

Tolerance and Physical Dependence Can Develop

For three classes of drugs, another factor contributes to the perpetuation and escalation of substance intake. All of the brain depressants, opiates, and stimulants described in Chapter 2 produce tolerance. This means that once use becomes fairly regular, in order to obtain a pleasant "high" and to develop levels of actual intoxication, higher doses of the drug are usually required. The more of the drug that is taken and the more regular the use, the higher become the doses that are required for an effect.

Furthermore, when the user reaches a relatively high level of frequency and amount of intake, the brain begins to change physically to try to fight the drug effects. These physical changes usually take weeks to develop for most drugs, although they can occur over a matter of days for the more potent stimulants. The alterations in brain functioning result in a condition where the body has changed so much that it cannot function normally unless the drug is available. This state of physical dependence (or physical addiction) then requires that the user take the substance on a regular basis to avoid feeling the type of withdrawal symptoms described in Chapter 3. This condition makes it far more difficult to quit permanently.

Before I go any further, some of you will be tempted to look at tolerance and physical dependence and say that because you don't have these problems you don't have a substance abuse problem. Not true! Remember that the essence of an alcohol or drug abuse problem is that you are willing to continue to take the substance despite the difficulties it causes. For the majority of substances, and for the majority of people who require help for their alcohol or drug problems, severe and impressive levels of tolerance and withdrawal never develop. Yet, a person can face terrible legal, health, interpersonal, and financial problems with a substance without ever developing physical addiction.

An Overview of the Process Through Some Examples

Perhaps some examples will help demonstrate the nature of substance abuse and dependence.

I have a dear friend who went through all of the stages of problems with alcohol described in this section but who never had severe alcohol withdrawal. She began with occasional use, had minor problems, including arguments with her husband and some blackouts where she forgot what had occurred during a drinking period. She then set rules for herself, demonstrated she could stop, had times of control, and yet would have unpredictable periods when the rules would fail her and the same difficulties would develop. She blamed all of the arguments in her marriage on her husband, the missed assignments at work on her boss, and the repeated accidents on bad luck. Despite these difficulties she was so competent and productive at work that even when producing at 50% of her optimal level, she never lost her job. At the same time, she was usually such a loving and caring wife and mother that the obvious deterioration in her marriage and distancing from her children never resulted in a separation or divorce. Unfortunately, it took the crisis created by her drunk-driving arrest (including being handcuffed and taken to jail for booking) to convince her husband that he could take no more. This episode *finally* precipitated a crisis that resulted in her agreeing to see a counselor to discuss her drinking problem.

The second case involves a highly successful physician I treated much earlier in my career. He began his use of codeine after breaking a leg in an auto accident and returned to the drug because of headaches related to the stress of work. As his opiate use escalated, he felt that his lack of sexual drive and emotional distancing from his wife were the results of her constant nagging, and he blamed his irritability at work on what he saw as the mistakes and inappropriate demands of his colleagues. Yet his competence, devotion to his family, and ability to make a good living insulated him from recognizing how severe his problems were until, eight years into his substance problem, the crisis hit. One weekend, while on call at a hospital, he "borrowed" codeine from the nurses' station. Caught almost "red-handed," he was referred to his chief of staff and subsequently to a "physician diversion" program for treatment. This is yet another example of a competent, caring, moral person for whom plenty of signs indicated that drug use meant more than the problems it was causing. Despite periods of abstinence and control, his use inevitably led to serious problems.

A final example focuses on an age group where drinking and alcohol-related life problems are very likely to be seen. Recently, I was asked to consult on the case of a sixteen-year-old boy whose parents feared that he had begun to develop more than the usual level of involvement with marijuana and alcohol. They were concerned because when he went from eighth to ninth grade, his grades dropped, he couldn't motivate himself to study or organize his homework, and he emotionally withdrew from the family. He developed mood swings that seemed out of proportion to what his parents had observed in other teenagers. The parents also noted that the young man seemed to reject friends who were better students and was almost exclusively associating with a group that partied a good deal and was likely to cut school.

As the story developed through repeated meetings with the young man, he related a history of perhaps six months of "casual" use of both alcohol and marijuana, during which he consumed levels that were consistent with most of his fellow students, even those who were getting good grades and appeared to have high levels of motivation. However, as his use of marijuana increased to four or five times a week along with heavy drinking at parties on weekends, he found himself getting into more verbal fights (and occasional physical fights) at school and at parties, admitted to taking money from his parents in order to "have a good time," and recognized that his grades were dropping rapidly. Despite these difficulties, he denied to himself that there were any *real* problems, feeling instead that his experiences were perfectly normal and no different from those of any other red-blooded adolescent. He tended to blame his poor grades on bad teachers, his choice of friends on rebellion against his parents' "ridiculous" high standards, and his fights and mild brushes with the law (as parties were broken up by the police) on bad luck. Although he has agreed to continue to see me (perhaps because he realizes that his problems are escalating, even though he is not willing to outwardly admit it), he is not yet willing to give up his peer group or his substance use pattern. However, as long as he is willing to continue to talk, I will continue to see him.

I hope the information offered in this section and these three brief examples give you some feeling about what substance use problems are like. The next section presents another important step for you to consider in evaluating whether a problem with drugs and/or alcohol exists.

If You're Trying to See if There Is a Problem, There Is No Room for Blame

By this point, you probably recognize that determining whether a problem exists requires some knowledge of the usual pattern of difficulties that develops in the course of substance problems. Because I don't know the specific history that concerns you, I have only covered generalities. Despite these more general comments, the key issue is to realize that if you have repeatedly returned to substance use even though that substance has caused a disruption in your life, you *do* have a problem.

I have already referred to a number of mechanisms that contribute to the development of substance-related problems. At least two of these processes, denial and a tendency to blame others, are so important to the perpetuation of the use of alcohol and drugs despite problems that they deserve mention in more detail.

The first problem is what is known as **denial,** a phenomenon mentioned earlier in this chapter. Denial plays an enormous and obvious role in substance abuse difficulties from early on in the process. After all, if the average substance abuser is no less moral or caring than the average person, when problems develop relating to substances, the individual must be denying something to him- or herself if he or she returns to substance use despite the problems. Although some people simply deny that the problems exist, most seem to insist to themselves that, although the problems are there, they could not possibly have been caused by the alcohol and drug usage. Often they cite the problems caused or made worse by alcohol or drugs as an excuse to continue to get high in order to cope. Yet others recognize the connection between life difficulties and their substance use, but they deny that the problems are important. Some others agree to the existence of difficulties but, despite prior experiences, are sure that this time they "can handle it." In any event, how could someone go back to the use of the substance after severe problems have developed unless he denied that the alcohol or drugs were causing the pain?

No one completely understands how denial works. The process occurs in all of us and is not necessarily bad in all situations. For example, the night before major surgery most of us would try to keep from our minds (deny) that what is about to occur the next morning could result in much pain and might even cause death. That very denial helps us to sleep on that night and keep our blood pressure down—protective steps that are likely to contribute to a more rapid postsurgical recovery. So, perhaps denial in substance use problems is in part a misfiring of a normal psychological defense mechanism, one each of us is likely to use in some situation or another. In any event, it is an essential component of the developing substance problems.

Another important contributor to continued substance use, one that is probably closely related to denial, is the tendency of the user to **blame** everyone and everything but the drugs or alcohol for the life problems he or she is experiencing. For example, if brain depressants such as alcohol are being used heavily and regularly, hangovers and mild levels of physical withdrawal often cause the user to feel intense nervousness, have problems sleeping, and even go into severe depression. Many substance users are tempted to cite these feelings (actually produced by the substances) as reasons to justify continued use. In effect, you are saying: "It's not my fault that I'm using drugs so much. If you were this depressed/anxious/tired/nervous you'd be using alcohol or drugs too."

Similarly, repeated use of stimulants, depressants, and opiates is likely to interfere with how well you communicate with others, produce periods of irritability, and eventually decrease your sex drive. All of these contribute to severe interpersonal difficulties. This is a big issue with even bigger consequences for you if you alienate friends and family. Thus, it is tempting (often almost irresistible) for the alcoholic or drug abuser to insist that he or she is taking drugs to help cope with that "son-of-a-bitch I have to live with" or to try to survive despite "those awful kids," or to learn to deal with those "rigid, demanding parents who obviously don't understand anything about me."

Perhaps one of the hardest things to get across to someone who is considering whether a substance problem exists is the fact that **there are truths of life for which blame is irrelevant.** The liver damage caused by alcohol and the crushed body after an accident are real regardless of reasons for drinking. Sorting out blame and determining who or what caused what condition does not change the fact that a decision to stop drinking or taking drugs must be made. The alcohol- or drug-related problems exist! The risk for severe illness or injury cannot be denied! And, the person involved with the substances is the primary individual who will really have to suffer when the consequences occur! How to get out of this situation is the most important issue.

A Note to Family and Friends

I hope the information presented here has helped you to decide whether the family member or friend you are concerned about has a problem with drugs or alcohol. In many ways it is easier for you to recognize substance abuse problems in other people than it is for the people with the substance problems to come to grips with their condition. This is especially likely when denial becomes a major obstacle to admitting a problem exists. Because you are more likely to be thinking clearly, it is probably more likely that you will be better able to evaluate realistically substance-related problems than the person who is drunk, high, or hungover for much of the time.

I also hope by this point you have learned that family turmoil and being blamed for the host of problems that accompany substance abuse is "par for the course." If humanly possible, it is a good idea to not take these attacks very personally, but rather to view them as a consequence of the drug or alcohol problem and the all-too-common tendency to blame others for difficulties.

Of course, as in any relationship, it is likely you did things that in retrospect only made matters worse. For example, you might have exploded in anger at being blamed for the substance abuser's problems, or you might have expressed your frustration at the user's continued denial of his or her life difficulties. These are often natural and understandable reactions that are likely to happen to almost anyone in a similar situation. However, as normal as they are, the reactions can sometimes make a difficult situation worse. These issues are discussed in greater depth in Chapter 11, and it might be worth briefly turning there to review that information now. In the interim, it is worthwhile to remind you that the first step to recovery is recognizing the problem, and it is only after sobriety has been achieved for a period of time that it will be possible for you and other friends and relatives to find out what the future holds for the relationship.

A Recap

Those of you who have an alcohol or drug problem, or have a relationship with someone who does, probably already had some inkling of most of the information offered in this chapter.

Substance abuse difficulties can affect anyone, and the crux of a serious drug or alcohol problem is that you are willing to continue to use these substances despite the problems they cause. These difficulties can include problems with the law, your significant relationships, with your health and safety, or with your school or work performance.

There is a strong and understandable tendency to deny some aspects of the existence of problems or the relationship between them and substance use. As human as this impulse is, a refusal to face the problems head on, no matter what additional life circumstances are involved, violates a rigid rule of nature from which no one can protect you: continued use *will* result in an escalation of problems, physical deterioration, and a definite heightened risk for an early death.

The next chapter speculates a bit more about how substance problems develop. Chapter 6 then begins the discussion of how these problems can be resolved.

References

1. Schuckit, M. A. Overview: Epidemiology of alcoholism. In Schuckit, M. A. (Ed). *Alcohol Patterns and Problems.* New Brunswick, New Jersey: Rutgers University Press, 1985, pp. 1–41.
2. Kozel, N. J., and Adams, E. H. Epidemiology of drug abuse: An overview. *Science* 234:970–974, 1986.

Additional Readings

Adlaf, E., Smart, R., and Walsh, G. Substance use and work disabilities among a general population sample. *The American Journal of Drug and Alcohol Abuse* 18:371–387, 1992.

Bucholz, K., Homin, S., and Helzer, J. When do alcoholics first discuss drinking problems? *Journal of Studies on Alcohol* 53:582–589, 1992.

Carroll, J. *The Basketball Diaries: Age 12–15.* Bolinas, CA: Tombouctou, 1978.

Dinwiddie, S., Rich, T., and Cloninger, R. Lifetime complications of drug use in intravenous drug users. *Journal of Substance Abuse Treatment* 4:13–18, 1992.

Helzer, J., Burnam, A., and McEvoy, L. Alcohol abuse and dependence. In: Robins, L., and Regier, D. *Psychiatric Disorders in America.* New York: The Free Press, 1991, pp. 81–115.

Kandel, D., Yamaguchi, K., and Zhen, K. Stages of progression in drug involvement from adolescence to adulthood. *Journal of Studies on Alcohol* 53:447–457, 1992.

Ludwig, A. Cognitive processes associated with "spontaneous" recovery from alcoholism. *Journal of Studies on Alcohol* 46:53–58, 1985.

Schuckit, M. A., Smith, T., Anthenelli, R., and Irwin, M. The clinical course of alcoholism in 636 male inpatients. *American Journal of Psychiatry* 150:786–792.

Skog, O., and Duckert, F. The development of alcoholics' and heavy drinkers' consumption: A longitudinal study. *Journal of Studies on Alcohol* 54:178–188, 1993.

Vaillant, G. *The Natural History of Alcoholism.* Cambridge, Massachusetts: Harvard University Press, 1983.

5

What Caused This Mess?

Goals

For some people, knowing that there is a problem is enough to make them avoid further consequences. Often, the reasons behind the difficulty don't matter—the question is what can be done to resolve the problem. For others, myself included, when something goes wrong in life, it helps to have some idea about what might have caused the problem. It is almost as if knowing more makes it feel as though we have some control or some say in what happens next.

This chapter reviews some theories about how repeated alcohol and drug problems might develop. I place a special emphasis on my own way of looking at things, but try to present a variety of theories, each of which contributes something to our understanding of what might be happening in substance use disorders. The decision to keep this chapter relatively brief is deliberate, because a true scholarly discussion of the pros and cons of the various approaches could fill an entire text in itself. While these debates are of great interest to some, they are not essential to anyone who is deciding whether a problem exists and what can be done about it. However, for those who want more information about the matters discussed here, some suggested additional readings are offered at the end of the chapter.

My Own Theory of Factors That Influence Use and Temporary Problems

The purpose of this chapter is to present some of the leading theories on factors that influence the initial decision to use a substance, those that impact on continued use despite minor problems, and those that might affect the progression from more minor, temporary problems to conditions of severe repeated difficulties that might be labeled as abuse or dependence. However, there is no single generally accepted theory that incorporates all of these three or more stages of potentially problematical substance use patterns. Therefore, one consequence of attempting to give a relatively balanced overview of different theories is that you might finish the chapter concluding that the issues are so complex that no general theory can be put together.

To avoid this problem, I've chosen to give you my own general theory first. Here, I begin with some thoughts on how social and interpersonal factors are likely to contribute to the choice to try a substance rather than remain abstinent for life. Once exposure to a substance has occurred, then a variety of other characteristics of an individual along with social and interpersonal influences contribute to the chances that substance-related problems are more or less likely to develop. However, many individuals with more minor problems learn from these experiences and stop or severely restrict use. Therefore, the third component of my own overall view of the progression of problems to the point of abuse or dependence focuses on those factors that combine to contribute to a relatively high risk for continued use despite more minor problems or, in other words, contribute to the development of abuse or dependence.

Some Thoughts on How Substance Use Begins

For most people, the willingness to experiment with alcohol or drugs probably reflects the attitudes of society, as well as the attitudes of close friends and relatives, toward the use of a substance. Here, when people around you indicate that it is acceptable to smoke, drink alcohol, or experiment with marijuana or other drugs, you are more likely to begin to use these substances than if your society and peers told you that such practices were fully unacceptable. Also reflecting society's attitudes toward substances, additional factors that contribute to the decision to experiment with a substance include relatively easy availability of the substance through, for example, a relatively low cost coupled with many sales outlets. The latter include the easy availability of alcohol and cigarettes through grocery and liquor stores, and the ease with which one can purchase marijuana or other illegal drugs in many large urban settings. Additional social attitudes can also contribute to the decision to begin using a substance. For example, the thought that smoking cigarettes is a step toward achieving an adult status is likely to encourage some individuals to begin use of this substance. Thus, for the majority of people, the decision to begin to use a substance (not necessarily to use heavily or to expose oneself to problems) is likely to reflect relatively common daily experiences, the attitudes of society, and the opinions of relatives and friends.

How Short-Term Problems Appear

Once a decision has been made to experiment with the use of a substance, a host of additional factors appear to influence the probability of developing temporary difficulties. The first of these factors is the nature of the particular drug being used. For example, difficulties are much more likely to be seen with even occasional use of the highly potent stimulants such as cocaine or amphetamines, as well as with intake of the more potent opiates such as heroin, Demerol (meperidine), and codeine. This is because these drugs can cause marked changes in your behavior the first time you use them, even at low doses.

With *all* drugs, no matter how powerful they are, a second factor that influences the risk of problems is how often you are likely to take the substance. Similar to the initial decision to use, this, in turn, is also affected by your attitudes and the practices of your friends. When a substantial number of your peers drink regularly, for example, it is more likely that you will become intoxicated on some occasions. The more frequently that happens, the greater the chance is that you will drive while intoxicated (as do perhaps one-third of people between twenty and thirty years old) (1). Frequent use also increases the chances that you will miss some time at school or work because of drinking (as do almost 40% of drinkers in their twenties), or that you will have an alcohol-related blackout (drinking so much that you forgot all or part of what happened during an evening—as experienced at some time by one-third or more of people who drink) (2).

Other factors, as we have said, that are likely to contribute to the chances you will take a drug frequently enough or in high enough doses to develop temporary problems include a low cost of the alcohol or drugs and their general availability. Most studies show that for alcohol (and probably for all other substances as well), any time there is a drop in the cost or increase in the number of sellers (including liquor stores or street dealers), more people will consume more alcohol or drugs (3). Other studies show that the more you use, the higher your rate of problems is likely to be (3).

Some Reasons Why Some Users "Progress" from Temporary to More Severe Difficulties

Up to this point, substance use and associated problems occur relatively infrequently. An additional set of influences is likely to interact to enhance the chances that more severe interpersonal arguments, more serious work- and school-related difficulties, and more complex medical and legal problems develop.

Almost every long-term study that has followed men and women over time has shown that *occasional* minor life problems from alcohol (and presumably from drugs) are not by themselves good predictors of severe future problems. In other words, whereas many people might experience temporary alcohol- or drug-related problems, these experiences do not necessarily mean that they will go on to develop more severe, persistent difficulties. However, for those people who do go on to develop serious, repeated problems (alcohol or drug dependence), there are a variety of complex forces that probably contribute to the escalation of their difficulties. These factors include: 1) the type of drug, since some substances like cocaine or heroin are much more likely to lead to higher doses and more serious consequences; 2) a person's biological reaction to the substance. For example, as discussed later in this chapter some people seem to require higher doses of alcohol to have even moderate effects. This encourages them to drink more, which then increases their risk for serious problems; 3) higher frequency of use, which for many drugs leads to tolerance as described in Chapter 1; 4) general life stresses, which might interfere with good judgment and make us feel that the effort to control use is hardly worthwhile; 5) the availability of the substance, and so on.

The factors that contribute to long-term difficulties are similar to those responsible for the appearance of *temporary* substance-related problems. However, since the majority of drinkers and those who experiment with other drugs never go on to develop repeated major difficulties, other factors must also contribute to the escalation of problems. Some of these additional factors are discussed in the next section.

An Overview of Studies of Factors That Might Contribute to Severe and Repeated Problems (Dependence)

It seems obvious that not everyone carries the same level of vulnerability to developing severe, repetitive problems once substance use has begun. This statement is really no different from what one would expect for most medical disorders, because different people appear to carry higher or lower levels of vulnerability toward heart attacks, cancer, obesity, and so on. Some people believe that different levels of vulnerability to developing alcohol or drug dependence are caused, at least in part, by biological differences that exist between people.

Some Genetic Factors Appear to Be Important

Most of my research over the last twenty years has focused on one important type of biological factor that might contribute to different levels of vulnerability toward developing severe substance-related problems. This is the possible role that *genetics* might play in the development of alcohol dependence or alcoholism. By this I mean the way in which the biological material or genes passed on from parents to children might predispose someone toward a higher or lower vulnerability to developing severe and repeated alcohol-related problems.

Unfortunately, there is less known about genetic influences relating to dependence on other substances such as the stimulants, marijuana-type drugs, or opiates, but even here new and interesting data are now being developed. However, since I want to keep my major emphasis on what is known (rather than what is guessed), I have to limit the comments offered here mostly to alcohol.

The fact that alcoholism runs strongly in families has been known for hundreds of years. Until relatively recently, however, most assumed that the twofold-to-fourfold increased risk for severe alcohol problems among close relatives of alcoholics was a result of the family environment in which people were raised. For example, it was assumed that a child raised in a home in which heavy drinking was the norm might learn that alcohol is a way to deal with problems. According to this theory, later in life such a person might be expected to develop more alcohol-related difficulties than someone raised in a home in which drunkenness was frowned upon and where alcohol was consumed in only moderate amounts or not at all. However, studies conducted in the 1960s began to question this presumption about the all-important role of environmental factors in producing alcoholism.

The first type of study to begin to test the relative importance of genetics versus childhood environment focused on twins. Here, researchers took advantage of the fact that nature produces two types of twins. **Fraternal twins** are born at the same time but share only 50% of their genes, the same as any full brothers and sisters. They come from different eggs and sperm, with two separate fertilized eggs being implanted in the womb at the same time. **Identical twins,** on the other hand, are also born at the same time but actually share 100% of their genes. They come from the same fertilized egg, which splits into two separate individuals after several divisions.

Both types of sets of twins are raised in the same environment and experience major childhood events at the same age and under the same general life conditions. Therefore, if severe alcohol-related life problems were the result of major events that occurred in childhood (i.e., environmental influences), then the twin of an alcoholic should have a very high risk for the disorder himself or herself, no matter whether fraternal or identical twinship is involved. On the other hand, if genetic factors are important, the identical twin of an alcoholic, sharing 100% of the genes, should be at a much higher risk for developing this problem than a fraternal twin. Almost all of the studies in this area carried out over the last twenty years show that the risk for alcoholism is much higher in the identical twin of an alcoholic (perhaps as high as 60%) than in the fraternal twins (with an estimated 30%) (4). These findings support the view that genetic factors play an important role in determining the risk for alcoholism.

To me, however, the most convincing evidence concerning the importance of genetic factors in alcoholism comes from studies of children of alcoholics who were adopted away close to birth. Here one can evaluate the risk for alcoholism among biological children of alcoholics who were raised by nonalcoholics. It is remarkable that these sons and daughters still demonstrate their fourfold increased risk for severe alcohol problems, even when they had no knowledge that their biological parent had had alcoholism. In fact, even if one of the children's adoptive parents develops alcoholism, this does not raise the alcoholism risk for the adopted child any further than what is predicted by the biological parent's problem. In other words, *a high risk for severe alcohol problems is predicted by the disorder in the biological parent, not by problems in the environment in which the child is raised.*

Genetic Factors Do Not Explain the Whole Picture

The discovery that alcoholism is influenced by genetic factors doesn't mean that genes alone cause severe alcohol problems. Some environmental factors must also play a role because the risk for the disorder in even the identical twin of an alcoholic is never as high as 100%. In other words, no one is predestined to become an alcoholic, anymore than anyone has a 100% chance for developing cancer or heart disease.

Thus, even if we have a higher risk for developing severe and persistent alcohol-related difficulties, we still have *choices* regarding what we do about it. We are the ones who decide whether we will drink at all, and we each determine the care we take to avoid drunkenness, the way we limit drinking at times of stress, and whether the development of more minor problems convinces us to avoid any use of alcohol in order to stop placing ourselves at risk.

Some Biological and Environmental Components that Increase the Alcoholism Risk Are Being Studied

A number of different research groups are now trying to find out how biological factors interact with the environment to contribute to the overall alcoholism risk. Some scientists believe that some aspects of the pattern of the electrical activity of the brain might indicate a higher alcoholism risk (5). This might relate to different levels of vulnerability to losing control of intake or to different vulnerabilities to brain damage. Perhaps these factors make some people more impulsive or make it harder for them to recognize when they are getting drunk. Other researchers think that the alcoholism risk might be related to genetically controlled enzyme systems and other proteins that might tie in to some personality characteristics (6). My own work raises another possibility.

Between 1978 and 1988 our research team studied 227 sons of severely impaired alcoholic fathers and another 227 young men (the control group) who had no known alcoholic biological relatives (7). We hypothesized that the sons of alcoholics were at higher risk for developing alcoholism later in their lives than the young men who came from nonalcoholic families. Both the sons of alcoholics and controls had already chosen to be drinkers, and this fact gave us the opportunity to evaluate how the two different groups reacted to alcohol. During what is called an alcohol challenge test, we asked all the young men to consume three to five drinks of alcohol, with the actual amount depending on how much they weighed. We found no differences between the sons of alcoholics and controls regarding how quickly the alcohol found its way into the bloodstream, the peak blood alcohol concentration that was reached, or the rate at which the alcohol disappeared from the blood.

However, despite the similarity in drinking history and the levels of alcohol in the blood, the sons of alcoholics showed less intense reactions to the alcohol they were given. This less intense response was observed in their self-reports of how they felt (the sons of alcoholics indicated they felt less "high"), in their levels of impairment in performing a task (with less loss of coordination in the sons of alcoholics), in lower intensities of changes in their brain waves, and in fewer alterations observed in some hormones known to change after alcohol intake. In other words, the alcohol had less of an effect on the sons of alcoholics than it did on the control group, so that the sons of alcoholics were much less impaired than the controls after consuming similar (but relatively low) amounts of alcohol. It is as if about half of the sons of alcoholics could "drink people under the table" from early in their drinking careers.

Yet, both the sons of alcoholics and controls reported to us that when they drank much higher levels of alcohol than we gave them, they were quite capable of becoming very intoxicated and impaired. Since the sons of alcoholics were able to function relatively well after three to five drinks, outside the laboratory in a social setting they might be predisposed to consume much higher amounts of alcohol than the control-group subjects. This is because the internal feelings after drinking for some children of alcoholics might not give them sufficient warning at the lower doses that it is time to stop drinking if heavy intoxication is to be avoided. We believe that this reduced sensitivity to lower doses of alcohol makes it more likely that excessive alcohol consumption and subsequent alcohol-related difficulties will occur in about half of the children of alcoholics.

The final step in our research is being carried out now. The same 454 men have all been located almost 10 years later (8). Interviews and blood tests are used to see who actually developed alcohol and other drug problems during the years following the initial testing. This allows us to see whether any of the original cognitive or thinking tests, personality measures, neurological evaluations, or evaluations of the intensity of response to alcohol predicted future problems with alcohol or other drugs.

So far the decreased reaction to alcohol observed among the sons of alcoholics *does* predict severe future alcohol problems. Among the sons of alcoholics, a very low level of response to alcohol at about age twenty was associated with almost a 60% risk of alcoholism by about age thirty. Sons of alcoholics with a high sensitivity to the alcohol challenge only had a 15% risk during the follow-up. On the other hand, we have not found that the family history of alcoholism or the lower intensity of response to alcohol predicts a high likelihood of developing severe problems with other types of drugs. A possible exception might occur for marijuana, for which there might be a slightly higher risk among children of alcoholics regardless of their response to the alcohol challenges.

In viewing this study, it is important to remember that we cannot perfectly predict who *will* become alcoholic. Nor can we even come close to telling who *won't* develop alcohol dependence. It is also important to remember that there are likely to be many ways to increase the risk other than the response to alcohol. However, it looks as if we might have uncovered one mechanism that interacts with environment to contribute to the alcoholism risk.

Contrary to What You Might Have Been Told, Most Alcoholics Do not Have Major Psychiatric Disorders

One theory that in prior years was often accepted by psychiatrists and psychologists stated that alcohol- and drug-related problems developed as part of a person's attempt to self-medicate major psychiatric problems. Thus, it was theorized that most alcohol- and drug-dependent people suffered from severe problems with anxiety, depression, or experienced symptoms of psychotic thinking, including hearing or seeing things that were not there or believing that people were plotting to harm them. These psychiatric conditions were theorized to have been present before the onset of severe alcohol or drug problems and to have significantly contributed toward the heavy use of alcohol and drugs in a futile attempt to control the psychiatric condition. However, the best data to date indicate that most people who develop serious alcohol or drug problems do *not* have a major psychiatric problem. In other words, for these people, alcoholism or drug problems are their **primary** disorder or complaint. As was discussed in Chapter 3, once anyone develops substance problems, he or she can be expected to have many psychological difficulties, including anxiety, depression, confusion, and psychotic symptoms (such as feeling people are "out to get them"). These symptoms can be a normal part of alcohol or drug intoxication or withdrawal. However, for people who do not have a major psychiatric disorder, these psychological difficulties are likely to disappear after a time following abstinence and the development of a lifestyle free of alcohol and drugs.

There are numerous studies that support this conclusion (9, 10). *First,* although 30% to 60% of alcohol- and drug-dependent people (especially those abusing stimulants and depressants) have very high levels of depression, anxiety, and high levels of psychotic symptoms when they come into treatment, these psychiatric problems usually disappear on their own with abstinence. If these psychiatric symptoms really indicated schizophrenia, major depressive disorders, or major anxiety disorders, the symptoms might improve a bit with abstinence, but would certainly not disappear. Several research laboratories have carefully evaluated depressive, anxiety, and psychotic symptoms in substance-dependent people. Here, the individuals were carefully observed and given general supportive care, but no specific medications or psychotherapy was aimed at the mood or psychotic problem. In 90% to 95% or more of these men and women, as predicted, the depression, anxiety, and psychotic symptoms (such as hearing voices or believing people were plotting against them) disappeared (9, 10).

A second type of study that supports the conclusion that most substance-dependent people do not have independent psychiatric disorders comes from observations of what happens to their children (7). If major psychiatric disorders were an important cause of subsequent alcohol and drug use disorders, then the children, who are at high risk for future alcohol and drug problems themselves, should show high levels of anxiety, depressive, and psychotic disorders *before* their problems with substances develop. Many different approaches have been used to evaluate this question, including studying both children of alcohol- and drug-dependent people as well as individuals from the general population prospectively over time. The conclusion from all of these studies is basically the same. There is no evidence that people who later go on to develop severe alcohol and drug problems are more likely than others in the general population to have had severe depressions, severe anxiety conditions, or psychotic conditions prior to the development of their alcohol and drug disorders.

A third type of study evaluating the relationship between psychiatric and substance use problems looks at the rate of alcoholism among men and women with psychiatric disorders, and vice versa (11). However, these studies are very complex because the evaluations have to carefully identify people who might only be showing temporary psychiatric symptoms while heavily using alcohol and drugs. When these considerations are added to the analyses, the general conclusions from these types of studies are that there is very little evidence supporting a high risk for a lifelong condition of a psychiatric disorder among alcohol- or drug-dependent people. Nor do the data support a high risk for true alcohol or drug dependence among individuals with major psychiatric disorders.

Finally, because most psychiatric disorders run in families, and because alcoholism and drug dependence tend to run in families, if alcoholism and psychiatric disorders were related, they should be seen in the same families. Obviously, this is not such a simple question to ask. All of the studies must carefully establish what they mean by psychiatric and substance use disorders. In addition, they must be certain that the illness in any relative of a subject might not just be the complication of alcohol or drug use. To make a long story short, a recent review of these studies did *not* demonstrate an exceptionally high rate of the co-occurrence of major substance use disorders and major psychiatric disorders in the same families (7).

For a Few People, Alcohol and Drug Problems Might Develop Because of a Prior Psychiatric Disorder

A small number of individuals with severe drug or alcohol problems also have a major psychiatric disorder. Unlike the majority of alcoholics and drug abusers, for these people, the psychiatric disorder is their *primary* problem, whereas the alcohol or drug problem is a *secondary* complaint. Individuals with a major psychiatric problem and severe alcohol or drug difficulties are usually easily identified. First, in most cases it is clear that the full psychiatric syndrome, not just isolated symptoms, predate the alcohol or drug problem. Second, unlike individuals for whom alcoholism or drug problems are the primary disorder, the psychological problems of individuals with major psychiatric disorders are likely to persist at very high intensities for months, even if those individuals give up their alcohol or drugs. However, there *are* three psychiatric disorders that are often associated with the later development of severe drug or alcohol difficulties. They are the antisocial personality disorder, schizophrenia, and mania. As described below, people suffering from one of these three disorders are at particular risk for developing serious problems with alcohol or drugs. However, most alcohol- and drug-dependent people do not have these preexisting disorders.

The Antisocial Personality Disorder

No one knows for sure where the antisocial personality disorder (ASPD) comes from. However, no matter what the causes might be, the antisocial personality disorder is a very dramatic syndrome that is fairly easy to spot before the development of severe alcohol and drug problems. Usually difficulties begin in the preteen years and involve major interpersonal and social problems that encompass *all* areas of life. For example, long before heavy involvement with substances begins, individuals with ASPD are likely to have problems getting along with their families and friends, and they are also likely to get into trouble at school and with the police.

The central problem with this disorder involves very poor self-control, and people with this syndrome often act on impulse to do or get things they want without regard for the law or the feelings of other people. Since individuals with ASPD find it difficult to feel sympathy for the rights and feelings of other people, they are often violent toward others who might "get in their way." This is often seen at age ten or twelve.

It makes sense that a problem with self-control and a lack of ability to feel sympathy or empathy for other people is often associated with a wide array of problems. For example, being highly impulsive and living in a society where alcohol and drugs are widely available makes it likely that alcohol or drug problems will develop as a consequence of this preexisting personality disorder.

Schizophrenia

About 1% of men and women in any society begin a slow progression of very disturbing psychiatric symptoms, usually starting in their teens to twenties (11). Here, the problems involve hearing voices that are not there (auditory hallucinations), thinking people are plotting against them, and a withdrawal from interacting with other people. Schizophrenia is a very serious, lifelong psychiatric disorder, and there are not enough long-term treatment facilities to take care of the needs of people with this syndrome. Because of this lack of social support, many individuals with schizophrenia are likely to be isolated and lonely, feel as though they do not fit into society, and spend a lot of time on the streets.

Perhaps as a consequence of their isolation, these people might be likely to experiment with alcohol or drugs. Probably reflecting poor judgment related to their schizophrenia, the alcohol and drug problems are likely to escalate quickly. It is also possible that, when taken in the early stages of schizophrenia when psychiatric symptoms can be quite mild, the use of alcohol or illegal drugs can cause a marked intensification of the psychiatric symptoms. It is important to remember that for this small proportion of alcoholics and drug dependent individuals, the psychiatric symptoms are usually apparent before the severe problems related to drugs appear. They are likely to remain permanently after drug use stops. However, people who only *develop* crazy thoughts or hallucinations *while using* substances, especially stimulants, do *not* have schizophrenia. In this case, the psychiatric symptoms are likely to disappear over several weeks to months.

Mania

This is a fairly rare psychiatric condition (also seen in about 1% of the population) that is characterized by severe and very incapacitating levels of excitement (12). Mania involves weeks on end when the person needs almost no sleep, feeling as if he or she has special powers, and these symptoms are often accompanied by thoughts that come and go so rapidly that it is almost impossible to control them. If this condition of mania is not treated properly, it can continue for months before it disappears. However, unlike schizophrenia, which is likely to be a lifelong chronic disorder, mania, and the periods of depression associated with it, are likely to occur as episodes that come and go. Between episodes, people are likely to be normal.

It should not be surprising that any disorder that causes bad judgment, high levels of impulsivity, and poor control over most behaviors is also likely to increase the possibility that alcohol and drugs will be taken in high doses. Thus, *during a manic episode,* substance problems are likely to develop. It is important to remember, however, that people who only become so hyperactive *while* using drugs such as the stimulants amphetamine or cocaine do *not* have mania. Those symptoms occurring with drugs are likely to be temporary and to disappear rapidly.

A Mini Recap

It is important to put this discussion into perspective. Remember that probably 70% or so of men and women with severe alcohol and drug problems do not have any major preexisting psychiatric disorder (7, 9). Many of these people can develop severe psychiatric symptoms while using drugs or alcohol, but these are likely to be temporary and to disappear on their own with abstinence.

However, when there is evidence that the antisocial personality disorder, schizophrenia, mania, or any other major psychiatric problem developed *before* the severe alcohol and drug problems began, this is an entirely different picture. These men and women *must* have treatment aimed at their psychiatric disorder, in addition to treatment for their substance use problem. Such people with primary psychiatric disorders and secondary alcohol or drug problems may have "gotten into this mess" because of the symptoms of their psychiatric illness. Another possibility is that they might have been unlucky enough to have concurrently developed two independent disorders, their psychiatric problem and substance dependence. After all, if at least 10% of men in the general population develop alcoholism, by chance alone at least 10% of schizophrenic men would be likely to have this disorder. No matter what condition came first, when there is evidence of an independent psychiatric problem, the treatment must consider all the conditions. *These are the people for whom psychiatric medications can be lifesaving.* Those who develop mania often require a prescription of the drug lithium, and treatment of schizophrenia often involves long-term use of drugs (including medications like Haldol or haloperidol) to help control the hallucinations and the paranoid thoughts. Here, the medications are not being used to treat the substance problem. They are, however, essential parts of treating the psychiatric disorder.

So, What Might All of This Mean to You?

The major impact of this chapter is to help individuals who are wrestling with trying to understand some of the causes of alcohol and drug dependence. As briefly stated earlier in this chapter, for some readers the causes are not a major concern, and, thus, a brief reading of the chapter will be sufficient. For others, however, it is important and often comforting to try to make sense out of a difficult situation. This requires that I offer more information about the influences that impact on the decision to use substances, those that contribute to more temporary problems (such as isolated alcohol-related blackouts, occasional driving or participating in other activities while intoxicated, and relatively minor arguments with family members and friends while intoxicated), situations that frequently convince the user that abstinence is the best future policy. It is important for some readers to try to understand more about how these early warning signs are not effective deterrents to everyone. So, information is also offered on those genetic, social, and other factors that seem to contribute to the transition from more occasional use with relatively rare problems to severe repeated life impairment from alcohol and drugs. The more intense difficulties include a break-up of a significant relationship, severe impairment in job and school performance, accidents related to alcohol use, evidence of physical problems resulting from substance use, and so on.

The present goal is to try to recap most of the major points made thus far in the chapter.

It is my guess that anyone who regularly takes alcohol or drugs in heavy doses is likely to develop *severe repetitive problems* with interpersonal relationships, job, and health. Social factors are likely to have a great deal to do with whether someone tries a drug, and a host of other influences, including the type of drug and the social setting, probably contribute to whether temporary problems occur. However, there appear to be some biological factors, including those influenced by genetics, that help determine whether a person experiments with a drug (including alcohol) and if such a use carries with it a heightened risk for repeated heavy use. Once the repeated intense exposure has occurred, then a combination of social, psychological, and physical factors develop to keep the substance use going. It is possible that the major difference between those who occasionally experiment with substances and "get away with it" and those who experience heavy enough use to develop problems may involve some biological and genetically influenced components.

Once a person is at a stage where he is using drugs heavily, a variety of social events usually help to perpetuate and even increase substance intake. For example, that person's light-drinking or non-drug-using friends are likely to fall away, leaving a peer group that consists mostly of heavier users. This increases the availability of the drug, and changes the person's view of what might be "normal" behavior regarding alcohol or drugs. The more of a substance you use, the less "abnormal" even higher doses appear to be.

At the same time, continued heavy use of any substance is likely to produce a level of psychological dependence (as described in Chapter 1) and lead to a feeling that the day is not complete unless the substance is taken. The more a person uses a drug, the greater the likelihood that a particular smell, a social setting, particular places, or the voice of a friend with whom drug use occurred will increase craving for the substance. It is as if our bodies and brains become "conditioned" to associate particular events with downing a drink or taking a drug. As substance use continues, the number of these associations increases, thus further predisposing us to more frequent intake of higher doses of the drugs.

The phenomenon of *tolerance* is another crucial factor, in addition to the social influences, that keeps substance use going once the individual has repeatedly used a substance. Tolerance is a relevant factor in continuing the use of depressant, opiate, and stimulant drugs. Tolerance occurs when recurrent intake of those three types of agents produces changes in the body as it tries to protect itself from the effects of the drug. Thus, higher and higher doses of a substance are required to cause the same effects. At the same time, for these three classes of substances, the body becomes unable to function normally without the substance, so that when the drug or alcohol is stopped, withdrawal symptoms develop. These body changes are part of physical dependence. These symptoms cause discomfort and pain, and the user soon discovers that these unpleasant conditions can be immediately relieved by taking some more of the drug. Obviously, once tolerance and physical dependence have developed, stopping use of the substance requires great effort and a high level of commitment.

These data and theories about the *interactions* of biological, environmental, and psychological factors discussed in this chapter help researchers to try to tease out characteristics that might be involved in causing the highest risk for substance use disorders. If we understand more about what helps to cause these problems, perhaps we can develop better ways to prevent them from occurring. Understanding about the complex nature of the interactions between substances and the people who use them might also help all of us to understand that not everyone with a substance use problem got there by traveling the same road. Therefore, there must be subgroups of people who might respond to different types of treatments. So, it should not be surprising that most treatment and prevention programs attempt to create aspects of the program that relate specifically to the needs of different patients.

It is important to emphasize some potential interpretations about substance use and problems that definitely are *not* valid. Some people look at the evidence for the biological component to substance use problems, particularly the data regarding alcoholism, and say that it means that they cannot help themselves—that they are predestined to develop problems with alcohol or drugs. If you accept this type of logic, then diabetics should feel predestined to an early death and give up their medications and special diets, and epileptics should feel excused from taking their medications and might consider themselves predestined to suffer consequences such as auto accidents caused by having a seizure while driving. Obviously, this is a ridiculous way to look at a predisposition toward a disorder. Rather, I view the biological component to alcoholism and drug abuse as an example of how, by bad luck and circumstances, some of us are more predisposed to developing serious substance-related difficulties than others.

However, a predisposition toward a disorder is not the same as predestination. No predestination is involved in alcohol or drug problems! Recognizing a heightened vulnerability to substance abuse difficulties gives a person the chance to escape the consequences. It should not be used as an excuse for allowing problems either to develop or to continue.

A Note to Family and Friends

The newspapers and some "pop psychology" books make a big thing out of a process called **codependence** (discussed in more detail in Chapter 9). Unfortunately, this concept has never been precisely defined. In its most acceptable form, codependence is taken to mean the actions, conversations, and behaviors of family members and friends as they interact with a loved one suffering from severe substance-related problems. This is how I use this term.

I recognize that living with an impaired individual is very difficult. I also recognize that friends and relatives don't always behave in the most rational ways, especially when they are under stress. When a relative or friend has a chronic disorder, including a substance use problem, everyone is likely to say and do things to decrease the tension in the house, to avoid a fight, to let out anger, and to try to survive under difficult circumstances.

If these interactions with the substance-dependent person go on long enough, the conversations are likely to become "scripted." Every time we smell alcohol or observe behaviors that we associate with drug taking, we get into the habit of saying "X," which our friend or relative responds to with "Y," which leads us to say "Z." And we are soon off to the races.

The optimal treatment for anyone with a chronic disorder requires reaching out to family members and friends. Treatment staff need to help you understand more about the nature of substance problems, assist you in making some important decisions regarding your own future, and teach you how to avoid (as much as possible) behaviors that might make the situation worse both for yourself and the person you love who is struggling with substance-related problems.

This chapter has focused on things that "caused the mess." I am certain that in every family there are actions and statements that might have contributed to the problem, or maybe even made matters worse. These forces, often listed under the umbrella of "codependency," need to be recognized and, whenever possible, dealt with. On the other hand, it is *very unlikely* that you actually caused the alcohol or drug dependence in your friend or relative. Recognition of the situation at hand and thoughts about how to minimize the likelihood of future problems are constructive; casting blame on family members is not only unproductive, it is often harmful. These comments complement the "Note to Family and Friends'' offered in Chapter 6. You might consider briefly turning to those pages now.

A Recap

This chapter began by asking how a person with substance-related problems got into this particular mess in the first place. If I have successfully put some of my thoughts in front of you, by this time in your reading you probably recognize how complicated a question this really is. The answer depends upon which mess you are talking about (substance use, temporary problems, or severe repetitive problems that might be called dependence), and which drugs are involved.

All substance use and subsequent problems relate on some level to **social factors.** These influence whether a person initially decides to drink or try marijuana or other drugs, and impact on the cost and availability of these substances. Social influences, including the attitudes and practices of friends, also influence how often someone takes a substance and that person's attitudes toward intoxication. Thus, social factors impact on use, temporary problems, and the vulnerability toward dependence.

Psychological forces also play an important role in this picture, especially in the development of temporary problems and dependence. In addition, for perhaps 20% or so of people with severe substance-related problems, their difficulties relate at least partially to a preexisting antisocial personality disorder, schizophrenia, manic depressive disease, or other psychiatric syndromes (7). For the majority of alcoholics and drug abusers who do not have major preexisting psychiatric disorders, it is likely that high levels of stress and some not very well-defined personality characteristics also contribute to temporary and more persisting substance-related problems.

Biological influences are obviously important in the development of problems related to the three classes of drugs for which tolerance and physical dependence are relevant (the depressants, stimulants, and opiates). Other biological influences seem to exert their effects through genetic mechanisms that markedly increase the chances that once exposed to repeated use of the substance some people have a high level of vulnerability toward escalating intake and subsequent persisting problems. Whereas the data supporting the importance of genetic influences for alcoholism are very strong, we can only speculate about the possibility that similar factors impact on a predisposition toward dependence on other drugs.

References

1. Klein, J. L., Anthenelli, R. M., Bacon, N., Smith, T., and Schuckit, M. Predictors of drinking and driving in healthy young men. *American Journal of Drug Alcohol Abuse* 20:223–235, 1994.
2. Anthenelli, R. M., Klein, J. L., Tsuang, J. W., Smith, T., and Schuckit, M. The prognostic importance of blackouts in young men. *Journal of Studies on Alcohol* 55:290–295, 1994.
3. Gerstin, D. Alcohol policy: Preventive options. In Grinspoon, L. (Ed.), *Psychiatric Update III.* Washington, D.C.: American Psychiatric Association Press, 1984, pp. 359–371.
4. Kendler, K. S., Heath, A. C., Neale, M. C., Kessler, R. C., and Eaves, L. J. A population-based twin study of alcoholism in women. *Journal of the American Medical Association* 268:1877–1882, 1992.
5. Begleiter, H. Potential biological markers in individuals at high risk for developing alcoholism. *Alcoholism: Clinical and Experimental Research* 12:488–493, 1988.
6. Tabakoff, B. Platelet enzyme activity in alcoholics. *New England Journal of Medicine* 318:134–139, 1988.
7. Schuckit, M. A. Low level of response to alcohol as a predictor of future alcoholism. *American Journal of Psychiatry* 151:184–189, 1994.
8. Schuckit, M. A. A clinical model of genetic influences on alcohol dependence. *Journal of Studies on Alcohol* 55:5–17, 1994.
9. Schuckit, M. A., and Hesselbrock, V. Alcohol dependence and anxiety disorders: What is the relationship? *American Journal of Psychiatry* 151:1723–1734, 1994.

10. Brown, S., and Schuckit, M. A. Changes in depression among abstinent alcoholics. *Journal of Studies on Alcohol* 49:412–417, 1988.
11. Goodwin, D. W., and Guze, S. B. *Psychiatric Diagnosis,* Fifth Edition. New York: Oxford University Press, 1994.
12. Schuckit, M. A. The clinical implications of primary diagnostic groups among alcoholics. *Archives of General Psychiatry* 42:1043–1049, 1985.

Additional Readings

Bickel, W., DeGrandpre, R., Hughes, J., and Higgins, S. Behavioral economics of drug self-administration. II. A unit-price analysis of cigarette smoking. *Journal of the Experimental Analysis of Behavior* 55:145–154, 1991.

Brown, S., Irwin, M., and Schuckit, M. A. Changes in anxiety among abstinent male alcoholics. *Journal of Studies on Alcohol* 52:55–61, 1991.

Committee on Opportunities in Drug Abuse Research. *Pathways of Addiction.* Washington, DC: National Academy Press, 1996.

Harrington, R., Fudge, H., Rutter, M., Pickles, A., and Hill, J. Adult outcome of childhood and adolescence depression. *Archives of General Psychiatry* 47:465–473, 1990.

Schuckit, M. A., and Smith, T. L. An 8-year follow-up of 450 sons of alcoholics and controls. *Archives of General Psychiatry* 53:303–310, 1996.

6

What Do I Do Now?

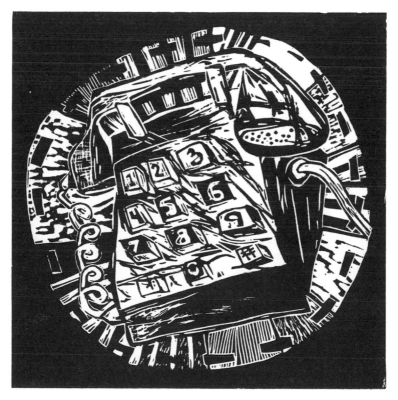

Figure 6.1. Once a problem is recognized, it is important to take action. There are many steps that can be taken to get help for yourself or for someone you care about. The first, and easiest, involves reaching for the telephone and calling the National Council on Alcoholism, a self-help group such as Alcoholics Anonymous, a treatment program that specializes in alcohol and drugs, a friend or trusted advisor, or anyone else that makes sense to you. The important message of this chapter is not to tell you which of the potential resources will work best for you, but to emphasize that any step toward recovery is an important accomplishment. Hopefully, after reading this chapter you will be ready to do something now!

Goals

If you turned to this chapter, you probably recognize that there is a problem and that something needs to be done about it. Because I recognize that some of you might also be reading this because someone you care about needs help, I have included a section directed at family members and friends.

Obviously, "getting out of it" is in many ways frightening. Once you recognize that there is a problem, finding your way out is complicated by an understandable fear that the price of quitting might be too high. You may fear that you will be forced to give up too many things in your life that are important to you. I hope that the discussion of these issues in this chapter will make it much easier for you to take a deep breath and take that first (and perhaps most important) step toward making things better.

What's There to Be Afraid Of?

People take alcohol and drugs for many different reasons, as discussed in the previous chapter. Many people like the taste, the feeling, and the rituals of substance taking. Most continue with substances as part of social interactions and find themselves selecting friends who share their views about alcohol and drug use. The thought of stopping raises many fears, some of which aren't even consciously recognized by the user as standing in the way. With these ideas in mind, I have listed some of the questions most people ask when considering giving up drugs or alcohol.

Couldn't I Just Cut Down?

Not only *can* you cut down, you *have probably taken this step* many times in the past. However, it is likely that no matter how many times you have been successful in cutting back on alcohol or drug intake, heavier use and associated problems always seem to crop up again. This indicates that, despite your best intentions, there is something interfering with your ability to control your intake of alcohol or drugs on a long-term basis. Whatever this thing is that makes control of your drug use difficult, it has nothing to do with an overall lack of self-control. However, the problems in the past certainly show that substances pose a real problem for you in the future.

By this point in your life, alcohol or drugs have become a central part of your lifestyle. So the thought of giving up something so important can be frightening. If there were any other rational alternative to abstinence, there is no question that I would recommend it.

Unfortunately, once a pattern of problems with a substance has developed, any use produces feelings of intoxication, feelings that decrease judgment and control. As emotionally wrenching as it is, for some reason, for you controlled use is only temporary and inevitably leads to additional problems.

So, there *is* a direct answer to the question. For people with past problems with substances, cutting down is almost always temporary and will certainly not solve the problems you face. You must stop all drug or alcohol intake to be sure to avoid substance-related difficulties in the future.

Couldn't I Just Give Up Drugs Temporarily?

The real problem here is that no one completely understands what causes some people to be more vulnerable to substance problems than others. As I discussed in the previous chapter, it is likely that there are a variety of factors that contribute to the risk, each working in a different way in different people. The end result is that if you have a heightened vulnerability toward substance use problems, no one can undo that level of high risk. It is there now, and it is always likely to remain.

This means that any time you decide to go back to substance use, you open the door to almost inevitable problems. On the other hand, the decision on how long you will avoid substances is totally up to you. Of course, stopping use for a week is better than continuing to take the drugs; stopping for a month is even better; and maintaining abstinence for a year is better yet. The longer you stay away from substances, the more you are likely to discover that there are many benefits to staying clean and sober. Perhaps you will even decide that the benefits of abstinence outweigh all of the things that you have given up by avoiding alcohol and drugs.

So, the answer to this question is actually yours to give. The decision to stay away from substances forever (and thus be sure of avoiding alcohol and drug problems) cannot be forced upon you. Furthermore, no decision is absolutely permanent, and you can always decide to go back to drugs or alcohol should you desire to do so. Returning to substance use is relatively easy. However, it is important that you realize that the longer you postpone abstinence, the more problems you will experience in the interim.

Can I Take the Pain of Withdrawal?

Let me reassure you about something. Although giving up any substance involves some psychological feelings (simply because you miss the drug and what it did for you), stopping most drugs does *not* involve life-threatening physical symptoms. For example, no obvious physical withdrawal symptoms are associated with stopping the use of marijuana-type drugs, hallucinogens (e.g., LSD), PCP, or solvents such as glue, toluene, or gasoline.

Physical withdrawal symptoms are only seen with three classes of drugs. These include the stimulants (such as cocaine and amphetamines) in all of their forms, the depressants (including alcohol and the Valium-type drugs), and the opiates (such as prescription pain pills like codeine, as well as heroin or methadone). More information about the withdrawal syndromes from drugs can be found in the readings for this chapter and for Chapter 1.

Those who have been taking increasing doses of any of these three classes of drugs (stimulants, depressants, or opiates) have probably actually gone through withdrawal many times. There is no reason to expect that this time will be worse than any of the others. For most people who use drugs that cause physical dependence, withdrawal symptoms begin within four to twelve hours of cutting down, are at their most severe on day one or two, and are well on their way to improving by day four or five. The only exceptions to this time course are the drugs that tend to stay around the body for a very long time, such as Valium, Librium, and methadone. Initial withdrawal symptoms associated with these long-acting drugs might not begin to develop for two weeks or so and might linger for about a month.

 It is possible to predict the types of withdrawal symptoms that might appear when you stop drugs. The physical withdrawal symptoms associated with these three classes of drugs are likely to be the opposite of what the drug did for you the first time you took it. For example, intoxication with *stimulants* involves having a lot of energy, not needing sleep, feeling as if life is wonderful, and a decreased appetite. Therefore, withdrawal, the opposite of these feelings, involves a lack of energy, feeling as if you have to sleep too much, symptoms of sadness and depression, as well as an increase in appetite. No prominent physical problems are likely to be experienced, and after approximately the second day of abstinence, the intensity of the symptoms becomes less and less.

 Intoxication with *depressants* is often accompanied by a feeling of relaxation, sleepiness, and several more subtle physical changes most of us don't pay much attention to (for example, a slight drop in the heart rate and body temperature). Therefore, withdrawal from alcohol, the Valium-type drugs, or the barbiturates (e.g., Seconal) involves insomnia, increased levels of nervousness, trembling of the hands, as well as slight increases in heart rate, breathing rate, blood pressure, and body temperature. While 95% to 98% of people only have mild-to-moderate withdrawal symptoms, perhaps 3% experience a convulsion or a state of mental confusion (1, 2). When these occur, this often means that there is some sort of medical problem that exists in addition to the substance problem.

The *opiate-type drugs* are all painkillers. During intoxication they produce prominent feelings of a floating sensation, a decrease in the perception of pain anywhere in the body, sleepiness, and a variety of physical changes in the lungs and digestive tract. Some of these changes explain why codeine can be so helpful in decreasing the symptoms of a cough, and why many opium-like drugs are helpful in treating diarrhea or abdominal pain. It should not be surprising, therefore, that withdrawal from these substances involves agitation, a magnification of any body pain, a runny nose and cough, as well as abdominal pain and diarrhea.

It has taken me a long time in this description to get to this point, but there *is* a direct answer to the question posed above. **For many drugs there is no withdrawal syndrome.** For others, not only can you stand the withdrawal symptoms, but it is likely that you have done so many times before. The very dramatic portrayal of withdrawal from alcohol or opiates seen in some movies is not what the average person goes through. In fact, many people think that withdrawal is actually one of the easiest steps on the road to developing a sober lifestyle.

Finally, the severity of the physical withdrawal symptoms I have described can be fairly easily minimized by a couple of measures. First, withdrawal from any of the three physicially addicting classes of drugs is best carried out under the supervision of a physician (even if on an outpatient basis). Your physician can give you a good physical exam, so you can be sure that you are not about to go through even mild withdrawal while physically impaired. Your doctor can also give you some education and reassure you that help is available. In addition, for two of the types of withdrawal that involve physical symptoms, those associated with depressants and opiates, there are medications available to lessen the discomfort of withdrawal.

Will I Be Able to Sleep without the Drug?

When you stop using drugs that are not physically addicting, there is no reason to expect physical symptoms that interfere with sleep. Furthermore, even if you have been using stimulants, which are physically addicting, you are likely to have too little energy and sleep too much during the first clean week.

The most significant problems with sleeping are likely to be seen after stopping the opiates and depressants. However, even here, the medications that are prescribed to help people through the first week of abstinence often produce sleepiness as a side effect and, thus, do help treat the sleep problems to some extent. Although sleep patterns are likely to return to normal soon after the first week or so of abstinence from opiates, the depressant drugs pose a longer-term problem regarding sleep.

Some level of interference with sleep can continue for a number of months after withdrawal from depressants, although the sleep pattern becomes more and more normal every week. Although there are no medications to help withdrawal-related sleep problems on a longer-term basis (i.e., after the first week or so of abstinence), there are some steps that can be taken to "retrain" the body to sleep more normally. This period of retraining might take as long as four weeks or so.

The *first step* involves getting up at the same time every day seven days a week. The *second step* is to establish a usual time of going to bed. However, remember to give yourself permission to read, watch television, watch a videotape, and so on if you do not fall asleep fairly quickly, for example in 15 minutes or so. The *third step*, one that is absolutely essential, is to take no naps during the day so that you can retrain the body that the only time for sleep is at night. *Fourth,* it is important to avoid any substances that might interfere with sleep, especially in the late afternoon or evening. This includes caffeine! *Finally,* and of equal importance with the other steps, is the need for you to recognize that if you have a restless night, as long as you don't nap during the next day and you avoid caffeine in the afternoon or evening, it is very likely that you will sleep much better the following night. Although sleeping problems may make you irritable and a bit frazzled, remember that lack of sleep won't kill you. Your sleeping problems are temporary and will almost certainly improve with continued abstinence.

So, in direct answer to the question, of course you will be able to sleep after you stop taking most types of drugs. For some of these substances (including the stimulants), during withdrawal you are likely to be sleeping a bit too much, and it will take you a while to get your energy back. Even for withdrawal from the depressants, which causes the most serious sleeping problems, the sleep impairment is only temporary and will improve fairly rapidly as time passes.

Will I Be Able to Handle X If I Stop?

That X is a "fill-in-the-blank." Some people continue to take drugs or alcohol because they believe they will not be able to cope with major life problems without the assistance of the substance. These problems might be related to a traumatic childhood or severe stress caused by painful war experiences. Others may fear that they will not be able to live with the discomfort of a bad back or another chronic pain syndrome, or that they cannot get over the loss of someone they loved without continued substance use. In many of these cases, the person believes that the life difficulty preceded the substance problem, and the person has become accustomed to the thought that the drugs are helping him or her cope. Other people may not have such serious preexisting life problems, but they share the belief that they need drugs or alcohol to get through the day.

However, this is simply not so! Most of the research evidence points to just the opposite. For example, almost all drugs cause mood swings. Thus, the emotional traumas you might forget about tonight as you are drunk or high become *many times* more difficult to deal with tomorrow when you are recovering from the effects of the drug. Similarly, physical pain might seem to improve as you take the alcohol or codeine, but the "rebound" (an increase in the amount of pain you have) that you experience tomorrow as you cut down on the drug may actually make the pain much worse. Finally, the life problems that you face with your spouse, relatives, children, boss, and others can hardly be handled when you are intoxicated (and not thinking clearly), or when you are experiencing mood swings related to almost any of the substances of abuse.

In addition, although many people don't like to admit it, many of the problems did not really exist before the substance use increased. Many of the difficulties are actually the *direct result* of the heavy intake of substances. Perhaps some examples will drive this point home. A number of years ago, a colleague and I carried out a study where we asked a large group of alcoholic women whether they believed that obstetric and gynecological difficulties had "caused" their alcohol problems (3). A majority of these women blamed their drinking on premenstrual tension, a spontaneous or induced abortion, menopause, difficulties during childbirth, and so on. However, when another interview and a search of hospital and other treatment records were carried out, it became clear that most of these women were kidding themselves. In the majority of these cases, the substance-related problems had developed long *before* the physical difficulty appeared. In many instances it also became apparent that heavy alcohol intake actually caused or contributed to the development of some of the obstetric or gynecological problems. Heavy drinking causes hormone changes that contribute to menstrual irregularities and increase the chances of having a spontaneous abortion.

Similar findings were also reported in a recent study of people who had both a chronic pain problem (e.g., a bad back) and severe substance difficulties (4). Reviews of treatment records and interviews with friends revealed that, contrary to the beliefs of the individuals involved, the substance problem was likely to have developed before the pain problem, not the other way around. In addition, the substance problem often had *contributed* to the injury that caused the chronic pain.

Another interesting case occurs with people who have symptoms of nervousness and depression, both of which are common among individuals with substance problems. Many people who abuse or are dependent on alcohol or drugs are convinced that their substance use helps them to cope with their pain or the nervous or depressed symptoms. In a way they are right. For example, people who take brain depressants like alcohol, or who use opiates on a regular basis, are likely to find that they wake up feeling very sick, nervous, or shaky every morning. They are probably aware that by taking alcohol or opiates they can make some of these unpleasant symptoms disappear. However, the symptoms that they are experiencing are likely to be the *result* of withdrawing overnight from the drug. In other words, the drug caused the symptoms of nervousness and shakiness in the first place. At this point, the person basically has two choices. He can decide to continue to take the drug, thus guaranteeing himself that almost every morning he will experience these same symptoms. The second choice is for him to acknowledge that the drugs themselves are contributing to the anxiety or the feeling of depression, and to take the first step toward getting off and staying off the substance use merry-go-round.

So there is a fairly direct answer to this question. YES, YOU CAN HANDLE PROBLEM X IF YOU STOP TAKING SUBSTANCES. For those of you with definite preexisting problems (such as a traumatic stress earlier in life), the mood swings, interference with thinking, and impairment in sleep that often accompany drug use are only making the nightmares and sadness or anxiety worse. You will be able to handle your life problems much more easily without the drugs—especially after several weeks of abstinence. Those of you without preexisting problems, but who are also suffering the consequences of heavy drug or alcohol use, will likewise find that you feel in better control and more able to make rational decisions when clean and sober.

I know you are likely to be in a difficult situation, and, believe me, I recognize that working your way through these problems is tough. I also realize that from where you are sitting, stopping substance use seems as if it will only make matters worse. However, every bit of medical experience I have (and the best data from the scientific literature back me up on this) suggests the only way to make these problems better is to stop taking substances and begin rebuilding your life.

I'll Be Humiliated!

Notice that this is a statement, not a question. Almost everybody who feels that some area of his or her life is out of control dreads the repercussions that may occur when they, in effect, admit to the world that a problem exists. Many fear that friends and co-workers will think they are weak, their children will not respect them, their spouses will no longer listen to them, or that it will be impossible to hold their heads up.

This is a very natural and understandable fear. But if you arrive at that conclusion, you ignore some important facts. Most people around you who didn't know of the problem do not necessarily need to be told that you are attending self-help meetings like AA or getting some type of more formal treatment. In fact, these more distant acquaintances probably have enough distractions and other concerns in their own lives that they would hardly notice that you are getting help. Also, most people don't really care that somebody "had an active problem." They are more likely to be concerned with existing problems and how they might interfere with their own lives.

It is also important not to kid yourself, and to recognize that the people who are close to you, as a consequence of that closeness, are likely to know that something is wrong. They might think that you're depressed, irrational, nervous, disorganized, or irritable. Or, they might realize that all of these symptoms are temporary and are related to your alcohol or drug use. Those who love you, or are otherwise close to you, are certainly not likely to lose respect for you if they learn you recognized that you were not functioning well and have taken steps to get rid of the problem. For example, it doesn't make sense that your children, who have learned to live with your social withdrawal, mood swings, and inconsistent behavior, would be upset to learn that these problems are not their fault, but rather the consequence of your substance problems.

In any event, most people who stop alcohol or other substance use are amazed when they find out how many people actually knew that something major was wrong. This includes many friends and relatives who suspected that the difficulties were related to alcohol or drugs. Similarly, it is sometimes hard to believe the number of family members and friends who love you enough to be proud and happy that you are willing to go through all of the work that is required to get rid of the problem.

Of course, some people will be lost to you. First, there are those people with whom you have been drinking regularly or taking drugs and for whom your attempt at abstinence is really very threatening. After all, if they were to admit that you have a problem and need to stop, and if they acknowledge that their own substance intake is as intense as yours, they would have to confront the fact that they themselves have a serious substance problem. Second, there are (unfortunately) people from whom you have grown distant or with whom such severe problems have developed that the relationship is unsalvageable. Continuing alcohol or drugs is certainly not going to reverse the estrangement from this second group of people—in fact, it can only make the breakup even more ugly and painful.

So, let me change the exclamation point used in the heading for this section to a question mark. Whereas it is never pleasant to admit that something is out of control, worrying about humiliation is pointless and counterproductive. Whatever damage has been done in relationships is done. Some friends will undoubtedly be lost to you, and some relationships have been damaged beyond repair. However, you should be optimistic about the support and enhanced respect you can expect from your close friends and family if you try to achieve abstinence and rebuild your life.

Do I Really Have to Stop ALL Drugs?

The central issue here is to recognize how important it is to avoid all situations that increase the chance that you will go back to alcohol or drugs. You have already learned how complex factors contribute to continued use and high levels of craving for substances. Therefore, when you use other substances, any of the old cues or feelings that you used to associate with substance intake will increase the chances that you will also think about taking the drug that has caused problems. This increased focus or craving for drugs caused by the use of other substances certainly makes it harder to stay clean and sober. A second important point is based on common sense. Anything that decreases your feelings of self-control, makes you confused, or increases feelings of impulsiveness will markedly increase the chances that you will return to using the alcohol or other drugs that caused the most problems.

These comments relate to using substances other than the major drug for which you are considering getting help. For those of you with cocaine problems, it is very likely that you took alcohol and marijuana along with your cocaine during a high, and many of you may have used alcohol or other depressant drugs to help you sleep or to "come down" the next day. Most people with marijuana problems use their drug along with alcohol. Those with problems with opiates almost always turn to other drugs to help modify the high or to help them cope when the drug they really want, such as heroin, is not available. Almost everyone uses combinations of different types of drugs. Therefore, if your major problem has been cocaine, even if you have never had a serious difficulty with alcohol, marijuana, or other drugs, exposure to substances that you used to take with the cocaine will almost certainly increase your craving for coke. At the same time, any high from alcohol, marijuana, or other substances will definitely decrease your feelings of self-control and make it more likely that you will go back to the drug that has already caused you so many problems.

In the final analysis, even if you never have had trouble with drugs other than, for example, cocaine, you are stacking the cards against yourself if you expose yourself to alcohol, the marijuana-type drugs, or almost any other intoxicating substance. This is not to say that you have a "certifiable" problem with the other substances. It simply reflects the fact that taking these substances will interfere with your ability to successfully stay clean and rebuild your life.

Be Honest with Yourself about Why It's So Hard to Stop

The next section tells you how to take that first step toward getting help. But before we get to that point, I want you to know that I understand you'll be giving up a great deal by stopping alcohol or drugs. I think it's important to recognize this fact because professionals offering help to people with drug or alcohol problems have a tendency to concentrate only on the consequences of substance use. We sometimes make it sound as though it's obvious that substances are "terrible" agents, and that anyone in his or her right mind would throw them straight out of the window or flush them down the toilet. We often forget how important alcohol or drugs have become in people's lives.

Everyone likes feeling good. When you have found a drug that temporarily helps you to feel more relaxed, gives you more energy, helps you to sleep, or decreases your physical and emotional pain when it makes you high, giving it up is like saying good-bye to a security blanket. This step is made even more difficult when past experience has shown you that when you stop using there are sometimes physical problems and certainly some levels of psychological craving that develop.

The advice offered in this text never ignores the fact that you have been taking substances because they supply you with something you want. Giving up friends who drink or use drugs heavily, avoiding social situations (including parties) where drugs are available and pushed, and saying good-bye to weekend binges is nothing you welcome.

That said, it is important for you to recognize that while you are now facing a difficult situation, it is not unique, and there are lots of parallels in life. For example, people with diabetes are not likely to stop loving pizza. However, they reach a point in their lives when their vulnerability to developing severe medical complications makes the price they pay for violating their strict diet too high. Similarly, the joyful eater who develops an allergy to lobster is likely to reach a point where he or she recognizes that the price of an allergic reaction is greater than the immediate benefits of tasting one favorite food.

Giving up substances of abuse does *not* mean you have to convince yourself that you did not like the drugs, alcohol, and associated good times. Of course you liked them, and it is definitely going to be a sacrifice to give them up. Much that you have read to this point, however, has taught you about the price that has to be paid if you continue to use. These adverse consequences are almost a law of nature: they are not your fault, they are not my fault. However, there's no way to avoid the problems as long as substance use continues. If you go back to alcohol or drugs, you will welcome back into your life an old friend, but the price to be paid is likely to be astounding.

To Begin, Pick a Step and Take It. Today!

It all seems so simple. Really, once the motivation is there, taking the first step *is* fairly straightforward. There are many ways to start, and the one that you select will be based on personal preference, past experiences, the resources presently available to you, the experiences of your friends, and your finances.

Before you pick up the phone or go to your first meeting, there are some things that you should keep in mind. It's a matter of luck as to whether the person on the other end of the phone line, or the first man or woman you bump into at a meeting, is in a good mood, speaks in terms that make you comfortable, or is competent to give you the advice that you are seeking. Neither you nor I can control those factors, so it is important to keep in mind that *if the first contact does not please you, that is not an excuse for giving up.* It often takes a series of exposures to different types of situations before you find the one that makes you feel comfortable. The beginning steps that you can consider include:

1. You can get information from the National Council on Alcoholism. Pick up your phone book, look in the *White Pages,* and call the number listed for the National Council on Alcoholism (NCA). It doesn't matter whether your problem is alcohol and/or drugs. All major cities in the United States have an NCA office where volunteers for this nonprofit organization will give you advice about the self-help groups and treatment programs available in your community. Just tell the person on the line that you are having a problem with X (fill in the blank) and want to learn more about what can be done. Ask them for a list of self-help groups (Alcoholics Anonymous, Cocaine Anonymous, Narcotics Anonymous, Pills Anonymous, and so on) in your neighborhood, as well as the names of some private practitioners or counselors and some treatment programs you might call to get more information. You risk nothing with this phone call. You do not even have to give your name. But you will be amazed at the number of programs that are open to you.

2. You can call a self-help group (Alcoholics Anonymous, Cocaine Anonymous, Narcotics Anonymous, Pills Anonymous, Rational Recovery), or stop in at a meeting. These organizations are all likely to be listed in both the *White* and *Yellow Pages* under "Alcohol" or "Drug Treatment." Although I cannot guarantee you will "like" or develop a rapport with the volunteer who answers the phone, I can promise you that this call involves no strings. All you have to do is ask about the meetings that occur in your neighborhood. In most big cities, there is likely to be a meeting somewhere near you every night of the week.

You can even ask the volunteer to steer you toward groups where you will feel most comfortable with other group members. Some meetings are mostly for men or mostly for women, whereas others have a good mix of the two sexes. Some meetings allow smoking, and others are for nonsmokers only. Some meetings are predominantly for white-collar workers, and others cater mainly to blue-collar workers. Furthermore, just as the membership of different self-help groups can vary, so too can the focus of group discussions. For example, some groups emphasize religion more than others, some tend to use readings and study groups, whereas others rely on verbal explanations of individuals' experiences with substances and the subsequent fight for recovery.

If you didn't like the first meeting you go to, try to figure out what it was that made you uncomfortable and find another meeting that offers more of what you are looking for. However, do not play the game with yourself that because you are not comfortable with one particular aspect of a meeting, or even one specific meeting, that self-help groups are not for you. There *will* be a program that meets your needs, if you take the time to look for it.

One final note about self-help groups deserves mention. Because part of the process of giving up substances almost always involves giving up any other situation that is likely to decrease motivation or stir up feelings closely associated with the actual use of the problematic substance, most people strongly advise you to give up all substances at the same time. Therefore, it is "kosher" for people with problems with codeine to join Alcoholics Anonymous, or for people with cocaine problems to feel more comfortable with the people that they meet at Narcotics Anonymous, and so on. The lines between these self-help groups are not rigidly drawn.

3. You can get information from a formal treatment program. You can use the *Yellow Pages*—looking under the headings Alcoholism Information and Treatment Centers, or Drug Abuse and Addiction Information and Treatment Centers—to locate an inpa-

tient or outpatient program. The counselors who do the phone screening are obligated (and often eager) to give you some information that allows you to begin to seek help. This should be true even if you do not eventually come to that specific program. Just call, explain that you are having a problem with X, and that you do not even know where to start to get help. Ask them for suggestions. Sometimes, it is even possible to arrange for a screening interview at no cost.

4. There are formal treatment programs to go to even if you have no insurance. Anyone who has served in the armed services and received an honorable discharge could be eligible for screening at an outpatient clinic or medical center run by the Department of Veterans Affairs (VA Hospitals). It is likely that these programs will soon be available for nonveterans as well. Veterans with relatively low incomes and individuals who received recognition of a service-connected disability are certainly eligible for formal treatment. Many of these programs are wonderful. At the very least, even if formal treatment isn't offered, important information could be obtained.

Some (not all) cities and counties have established low-cost formal treatment programs for mental health problems such as depression or anxiety and/or for alcohol or other substance difficulties. Going through screening frequently involves paperwork and red tape, steps that are likely to guarantee an evaluation but not necessarily deliver formal treatment. If, for some reason, the steps offered above did not work for you, there is little to be lost trying this route. A good place to start is the "Government Pages" of the *White Pages* phone book; look for listings under "Alcohol," "Drugs," or "Crisis."

5. Some other resources are also available. Carrying a professional degree does not, by itself, guarantee expertise about identifying and treating substance-related problems. So, I cannot promise you that asking your physician or pastor about substance problems and appropriate treatment will result in useful information or actual help. On the other hand, these are generally promising resources because greater and greater numbers of these pro-

fessionals are receiving special training in substance-related problems.

A Note to Family and Friends

If you have been reading this chapter in hopes of learning how to help someone you care for begin to take steps to address his or her substance problems, all of the information offered above has some relevance. However, you might also face the difficulty of trying to decide what to do if the person you care for refuses to seek help.

First, both the National Council on Alcoholism and the self-help groups like Alcoholics Anonymous are as much for families and friends as for the person with the substance use difficulty. For example, a telephone call to AA can identify groups for family members, called Alanon, and special groups for children, called Alateen. These are places where people can go at no cost to learn more about important decisions that have to be made when one is close to someone with alcohol or drug problems. You will have the opportunity to learn how other people have set their own priorities and recognize that you are not alone in what you feel. Remember that most people who come to these meetings have no alcohol or drug problems themselves. They are there to learn about what options they face regarding their friend or loved one.

One of the things you are likely to learn in any of these self-help groups can briefly be discussed here. If your goal is to try to help your family member or friend to recognize the problems that substances are causing and to maximize his or her motivation to do something about it, there is a difficult but important step you must take. *This step requires a commitment on your part to stop doing anything that protects the person from the consequences of his or her substance abuse.* For example, don't "call in sick" to work or school for the person with problems, don't rescue the person from jail in the middle of the night, and don't help the individual up to bed if he or she has thrown up in the bathroom or fallen asleep on the floor. It makes sense that if stopping is so hard and if drugs or alcohol means so very much to the person, unless that person comes nose-to-nose with the consequences of his or her substance use, he or she will find it very difficult to gather up enough energy to take the steps necessary to quit.

Furthermore, no matter how much you love and care for the person with a substance problem, you cannot "rescue" him or her. If you care, your job is to do everything possible to maximize the chances that he or she will seek help and stop substance use. The decision to stop rests totally with the drug- or alcohol-dependent person, not you. If you push too hard, you are falling into the game of "Make Me Do It." Shy of hog-tying substance-dependent people and physically carrying them to the program (which is not only illegal but also unlikely to result in any level of cooperation), it really is not possible for you to make them do anything. If you do take responsibility for their actions, if you see it as within your power to make them stop, they will not assume this responsibility themselves, and their chances of achieving abstinence are close to zero.

Despite that caution, there are some positive steps that you can take. These are best done after you've learned something about substance use problems through books such as this, as well as through self-help groups. The essence of what you are trying to learn is actually an interpersonal skill, one for which only general guidelines (not specific cookbook-type rules) can be offered. The skill is called **confrontation.** Actually, this is an unfortunate name because it implies that there will be an adversarial relationship. The process would be better termed as a development of **increasing awareness** or **intervention.**

Even though I cannot tell you specifically how *you* should do it, I can give some general guidelines to follow if a family member or friend has serious drug or alcohol problems. *First,* bring up the subject of substance problems at a time when the person is neither intoxicated nor extremely irritable as a result of recent intoxication. The best times are actually when the individual is feeling fairly good and/or experiencing some remorse about how his or her life is going. *Second,* begin the conversation by admitting several things. These include the facts that you care very much about what happens to this individual; that you recognize that life decisions for him or her don't rest with you; and that you fully acknowledge that it is not your place (or within your power) to make anyone do anything. *Third,* you would tell the person that you feel that alcohol or drugs are having a significant detrimental impact on *very specific* life areas. The examples used must be more precise than "drugs are killing you." The best way to help people recognize the price they are paying for substance use is to cite specific events that occurred and the exact day they were observed. You might then focus on some of the person's more recent and dramatic life problems and point out the relationship between substance use and the particular life problems in question.

In the *fourth* step of intervention, you might tell the person that if he or she is ready to talk with somebody who knows more about alcohol or drugs than you do, you have the relevant names and telephone numbers and/or have arranged for an appointment. This means that you have to have done your homework before the intervention and recognize that if your discussion has occurred at 4:00 P.M., you know of an open AA meeting that begins at 6:00 P.M. and/or you've arranged for an appointment at 7:30 P.M. at a local program or with a physician/pastor, etc. *Fifth,* no matter how tempting it might be to expand this conversation to additional related topics such as general financial difficulties or problems you might be having with your children or in-laws, force yourself to focus on how much you care for the person and the specific manner in which the drug or alcohol has impaired his or her life functioning.

Finally, you might remind yourself that the word intervention should actually be plural. It is rare that one discussion results in a dramatic change in someone's life. So, if on this particular occasion your family member or friend denies the problem or refuses to seek help, you can look for another opportunity to bring up the problem again and to address the need to do something about it. You should continue to do this until either the relationship becomes intolerable for you or the person finally decides to seek help.

A Recap

It is hard to pick any one chapter in this text and say that it is the "key" to recovery. For example, if you don't understand enough about what drugs are and their dangers, it's hard to make an informed decision about stopping. Similarly, a lack of understanding about the complex factors that contribute to the development and perpetuation of problems can make it difficult to figure out how to escape. On the other hand, these issues are all a prelude to getting the motivation to take that essential first step and to begin to seek help. Once that first move has been made, the material discussed in the next chapter on how to select a more formal program flows naturally.

Therefore, I do consider the information offered in this chapter to be one of the key steps for you in getting something done about your substance-related life difficulties. I hope that I have shown that the physical and psychological consequences of stopping are not so awesome and have shared with you my understanding about how much of your life is likely to be given up with the drug. I hope that by this point you are tempted to take some of these first suggested steps. After making that first phone call or attending a self-help group meeting, you may be ready for the information offered in Chapter 7.

References

1. Schuckit, M. A., Smith, T., Anthenelli, R., and Irwin, M. Clinical course of alcoholism in 636 male inpatients. *American Journal of Psychiatry* 150:786–792, 1993.
2. Sellers, E. Characteristics of DSM-III-R criteria for uncomplicated alco-

hol withdrawal episodes. *Archives of General Psychiatry* 48:442–447, 1991.
3. Morrissey, E., and Schuckit, M. A. Stressful life events and alcoholism in women seen in a detoxification center. *Journal of Studies on Alcohol* 39:1559–1576, 1978.
4. Atkinson, J., Slater, M., Patterson, T., Grant, I., and Garfin, S. Prevalence, onset, and risk of psychiatric disorders in men with chronic and low back pain: A controlled study. *Pain* 45:111–121, 1991.

Additional Readings

Ancoli-Israel, S. *All I Want Is a Good Night's Sleep*. St. Louis: Mosby, 1996.
Schuckit, M. A. Treatment of alcoholism in office and outpatient settings. In: Mendelson, J. H., and Mello, N. K. (Eds.). *Medical Diagnosis and Treatment of Alcoholism*. New York: McGraw-Hill, 1992, pp. 363–392.

References for Family and Friends

Al-Anon Family Groups. *From Survival to Recovery: Growing Up in an Alcoholic Home*. New York: Al-Anon, 1994.
Galanter, M. Network therapy for addiction: A model for office practice. *American Journal of Psychiatry* 150:28–36, 1993.
Galanter, M., Gleaton, T., Marcus, C., and McMillen, J. Self-help groups for parents of young drug and alcohol abusers. *American Journal of Psychiatry* 141:889–891, 1984.
Galanter, M., Castaneda, R., and Ferman, J. Substance abuse among general psychiatric patients: Place of presentation, diagnosis, and treatment. *American Journal of Drug and Alcohol Abuse* 14:211–235, 1988.

Johnson, D. E. *Intervention: How to Help Someone Who Doesn't Want Help.* Minneapolis: Johnson Institute Books, 1986.

Kaufman, E. *Help At Last: A Complete Guide to Coping with Chemically Dependent Men.* New York: Gardner Press, 1991.

7

How Do I Find the "Right" Program?

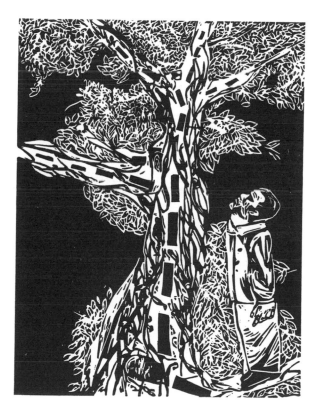

Figure 7.1. There are many different paths to recovery. Your choice of turning left, right, or going straight ahead as you are growing and learning more about the various treatment options available to you will be the result of relatively simple influences. You may choose a program because it is in your community, your health care provider feels comfortable with the program, or your insurance or health maintenance organization has a contract with them. A program might be more attractive to you because it offers specific medical facilities that you require or, perhaps, has staff members who are comfortable working with the types of emotional difficulties you might now be facing. There are influences, such as more severe social, medical, or emotional problems, that would argue for inpatient versus outpatient rehabilitation. In any event, this illustration demonstrates that no one road is likely to be wrong and the others right. No matter which program you choose, if you work carefully with the staff and recognize the need for continued support over a long period of time, you are likely to do quite well.

Goals

The aim of this chapter is to give you practical information to help you choose a program. The process of finding help involves trying to match your own needs and preferences to the huge number of potential programs available to you, so you can get help in a way that makes you most comfortable. The good news is that there are very few harmful or useless treatment programs for substance use disorders. In fact, most of the types of treatments for most of the forms of substances have very similar methods and goals, differing basically on how they get the job done and the physical setting in which they work.

A second bit of good news is that none of the decisions you are about to make is irreversible. You may need to "try on for size" a number of different approaches. Just remember that you will always have the option of rejecting the ones that seem to make little sense for your own needs. "Shopping around" is a good description of the process of finding the right program for you.

This chapter takes a look at some of the questions you are probably asking yourself right now. First of all, there is a review of the pros and cons of outpatient versus inpatient treatments. Basically, **outpatient** treatment means that you sleep at home and visit a facility to receive the care you need. **Inpatient** treatment, on the other hand, means that you actually stay at a facility for a period of time (usually during the most intensive first phase of your recovery). For both the outpatient and inpatient modes of treatment, there is a discussion of how to select a specific program that suits your needs.

Before beginning, I want to reassure you that there is no magical or single best answer to the problems you are now facing. In general, if you are highly motivated, then you are likely to do well in almost any program you choose. I also want to emphasize that some of the influences that are likely to help you to choose a program are already in place. These include the preferences of the friends or professionals with whom you have been dealing to this point, your family, the city where you live, and your financial situation.

Why Doesn't Everyone Select Outpatient Treatment?

Outpatient Care Has Benefits but Is Not for Everyone

As discussed above, outpatient care means that you sleep in your own home and visit the treatment program to receive care. Although you might imagine that everyone would prefer the familiar surroundings and comforts of home to staying in a residential facility, this treatment approach is not appropriate for everyone (see Figure 7.2). Inpatient care may make more sense in the following situations:

1. If you have *already tried* outpatient treatment, and it did not seem to work, it makes sense that some sort of more intensive and concentrated inpatient therapy would be a logical choice.
2. If you have moderately severe *medical problems* that require more than the usual outpatient attention, inpatient therapy might make sense. These medical conditions include substance-related heart problems, liver problems, infections, and so on.
3. If the levels of *depression, anxiety, or confusion* that are so often associated with abuse of alcohol and other drugs are so intense that you can hardly function on a day-to-day basis, inpatient care makes more sense.
4. If you are facing a *home or social situation* that is so chaotic that you feel unable to survive without greater support, inpatient care might be needed.
5. If you live in a setting that is so *far away from a treatment program* that you cannot regularly attend meetings, you might consider inpatient care.

At the same time, outpatient treatment *does* offer a number of important advantages. One of these assets is the substantially lower cost involved when the program does not have to pay for a bed and three meals a day, as well as around-the-clock nursing and physician care. Outpatient therapy also gives you the financial benefit of not having to take leave from your job. Finally, outpatient treatment means that you are receiving care while living in the "real world." In other words, you can learn to work through life adjustments while still functioning in your real-life situations.

So, the choice of inpatient versus outpatient care reflects a large number of options and considerations. I can't say that inpatient treatment should never be used because it is too costly or that outpatient care should always be avoided because it's not intense enough. The decision about which of these two general approaches is best depends upon all of the diverse factors I have just discussed.

If You Have Selected the Outpatient Route, to Whom Can You Turn?

It should not be surprising that there are a variety of different types of nonresidential therapies available to you. After all, look at the range of options that you could consider in choosing a particular dentist, a physician, an exercise program, and so on.

One consideration is the type of person you want to work with. For example, many physicians have set up private-practice programs where they treat men and women with substance problems in either an individual or a group setting. Similarly, other health professionals, including psychiatrists (physicians who have specialized in treating psychiatric difficulties), psychologists, social workers, and people with a host of different types of counseling degrees also offer possible outpatient care. A useful place to look is in the phone book, where many cities have listings under "Alcohol" or "Drugs," or by the specific training of these professionals, such as "Physicians" or "Physician Psychiatrists."

An even better way to begin is to ask for some suggestions from the people who helped you realize that you have a substance problem. Therefore, a call to the National Council on Alcoholism, any relevant self-help group, or an established treatment program, each of which is listed in the phone book, makes sense. You could also attempt to find an experienced counselor through your place of worship, work, or your school.

How Do You Find an Established Outpatient Program?

It is sometimes less costly to search out an established program rather than a specific counselor. Here, you can begin by looking in the *Yellow Pages* under "Alcohol" or "Drugs," or turn to the *White Pages* under National Council on Alcoholism (NCA), Alcoholics Anonymous (AA), Cocaine Anonymous (CA), Narcotics Anonymous (NA), or Pills Anonymous (PA). A telephone volunteer at any of those numbers can tell you about the outpatient programs in your community.

Once you have found a program that looks promising, the facility will almost certainly have an initial screening and then assign you to appropriate groups. For most programs, these groups will meet several times a week for up to a month, followed by a less intensive schedule likely to continue for several months to perhaps a year. All the formal outpatient programs I know of also offer important help in evaluating your job needs, in reaching out to family members and friends, and in emphasizing the importance of working with self-help groups such as AA, NA, and CA.

Several low-cost (and sometimes free) options can be found. For example, veterans of the armed services—especially those who have relatively low incomes, those with official service-connected disabilities, and retired career personnel—can approach their local Veterans Affairs (VA) Medical Center. Although there is often some red tape, the long lines and waiting are worth it. Despite the low cost, these programs are often excellent, and they compare favorably with many of the programs offered by the private sector.

Other people lacking funds can sometimes look to city or county mental health programs. Additional potential resources include some churches, religious-affiliated organizations such as missions, and a few independent groups like the Salvation Army or Goodwill.

When Inpatient Treatment Makes Sense, How Do I Choose a Specific Program?

As discussed in the prior section, inpatient care is not appropriate for everyone. The selection of this more intense and costly approach is often based on the severity of your medical, psychiatric, and social problems, your prior experiences with outpatient care, and your personal preferences. Some of the reasons why a person might consider inpatient care are outlined in Figure 7.2. These include having tried an outpatient approach that didn't work, or such severe medical, emotional, or social problems that the person fears he or she can't function on a day-to-day basis.

One important point to remember is that there is no evidence that inpatient treatment is always more effective than outpatient care. In fact, most studies that have compared the two approaches

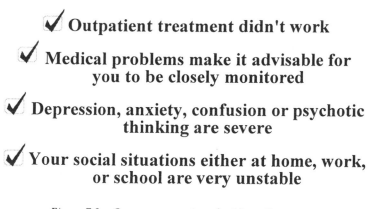

☑ **Outpatient treatment didn't work**

☑ **Medical problems make it advisable for you to be closely monitored**

☑ **Depression, anxiety, confusion or psychotic thinking are severe**

☑ **Your social situations either at home, work, or school are very unstable**

Figure 7.2. Some reasons to select inpatient care.

have found few differences in the levels of functioning of people six to twelve months after inpatient as compared to outpatient treatment. On the other hand, studies also show that some people who did not benefit much from outpatient therapies seemed to do much better after inpatient care.

Once the decision has been made to seek inpatient care, there are still many things to consider that impact on which specific program might best fit your needs. These are listed below.

The "Orientation" of the Program

Some treatment efforts take place in general medical and surgical hospitals, and others in psychiatric facilities. Additional programs can be found in "free-standing" buildings that are not attached to a formal hospital or clinic, and others are located in out-of-the-way places in rural settings. Which one should you pick? As you have surely guessed by now, the answer is "it all depends."

If you have medical or psychiatric problems as part of your substance pattern, even if they are not severe enough to justify an inpatient medical or psychiatric hospitalization, they can be part of the considerations used in choosing a program housed in a medical or psychiatric facility. When these problems are not part of the picture, some sort of "free-standing" program would make sense. This is because the absence of the resources that are part of general medical and psychiatric care often means that free-standing programs have lower costs and perhaps more staff available specifically to help with the substance problems.

Financial Considerations

As is true of almost all areas of life, some factors influencing your choice of a treatment program are likely to be beyond your control. Your financial situation and the nature of your health insurance coverage (if any) are two such factors.

For instance, you may find you are required to go to a specific treatment program as part of an arrangement made between your employer and its health insurance carrier. Often, the people or institution picking up the tab for the care will decide on a particular treatment program because its prices compare favorably with other similar programs. However, since most respectable treatment approaches tend to have similar success rates for the same types of people, such a lack of choice is not likely to have any major impact on the eventual outcome.

Recognizing that inpatient rehabilitation often costs up to $8,000 and $15,000 for a program of one to three weeks, lack of insurance can be a severe stumbling block in finding a suitable treatment program. Although some states have relatively low-cost inpatient care available (this was true of the state of Washington in the late 1970s), others offer few choices in the lower-cost range. Here again, however, veterans can reap the benefits of their service, since over eighty VA hospitals have inpatient alcohol and drug rehabilitation programs. The majority of these programs offer care comparable to (and I believe sometimes superior to) some private-care programs.

The Importance of Location

In addition to the type of facility—a general hospital, psychiatric hospital, or free-standing facility—the geography of the program is another important consideration. Here, I have a relatively strong bias based on my understanding of the long-term commitment required for the effective treatment of alcohol and drug problems. Remember that recognizing that a problem is present, and deciding to seek treatment, are only the first steps. Detoxification (treatment for drug withdrawal), when needed, is relatively short-term and straightforward, and all inpatient and outpatient programs focus most intensively on the first month or so of care. However, the *real work* is learning how to readjust to a lifestyle without substances, and this takes many, many months. The need for a long-term commitment to functioning without substances is the focus of Chapter 10. However, this issue can have a major impact on the decision of where to get treated.

The first, and most important, rule of thumb here is to choose a program in your community so that you can continue in aftercare for three to twelve months after the formal or intensive phase of therapy has ended. It is so much easier to deal with outpatient aftercare groups when you are already comfortable with the philosophy of the program and feel as if the counselors are old friends, almost family. In other words, it is helpful to get aftercare from the same group that gave the more intensive earlier stages of treatment. The selection of a program in your own community also allows family members and friends to learn more about substance problems and the process of recovery. Therefore, whenever possible, it is important to select a treatment program in your own community.

I know that this poses a problem for some people. An example of those facing such a dilemma are those people who are sent to an inpatient facility many miles from home as part of an arrangement made with their school, workplace, or an insurance company. Here, all is not lost. Rather, this means that extra efforts must be made while working with the inpatient facility to find an appropriate aftercare group and self-help organization such as AA. In this case, it is *very important* that you strongly encourage (maybe even force) the inpatient facility to help you, long before discharge, to set up appropriate aftercare meetings, giving you the opportunity to visit meetings while on passes before actually leaving the inpatient facility.

Another consideration many people have in selecting the geographic location of a facility rests with their fear of being embarrassed if they are treated in their home community. People who are especially well-known or prominent within their area may be particularly reluctant to have friends know about their problem. As I pointed out in the previous chapter, however, although this argument sounds reasonable (and sometimes might actually be appropriate), it usually makes less sense than we think.

This is because almost all family members and friends (at least any that are close to us) probably already know there is a problem. Even more distant friends are soon likely to recognize that your behavior has changed remarkably for the better and that your use of alcohol and other substances has stopped. It is also highly likely that the more people who know about your decision to abstain, the easier it is to stay clean and sober. It is almost as if by letting them know, you have made a direct statement that you are taking steps to make things better.

In any event, getting treatment near where you live is a very good idea. If you have to go away for care, however, you'll have to work extra hard to get aftercare and self-help group support set up near home *before* you leave formal treatment.

The Length of Commitment

The "commitment" to changing a lifestyle is yours—nobody else's. What I am referring to here is a choice you face about the length of your more intensive inpatient or early-phase outpatient care.

This is a good time for me to remind you once again that the recovery process from alcohol and drugs is measured in *months and years.* The steps involve the recognition of a problem, getting inpatient or outpatient treatment and rehabilitation, and then the real work. The latter, of course, includes aftercare and self-help groups that are important for the many months it takes to optimize commitment to abstinence and to rebuild your life without substances. In such a long and intense process, the choice of whether inpatient rehabilitation is ten days or four weeks is rarely a life-or-death decision. That statement is offered by way of reassurance. If either your own finances or those of the institution picking up the bill for inpatient rehabilitation mean that you go to a two-week rather than a four-week inpatient program, that is not necessarily a bad thing.

Most inpatient rehabilitation efforts offer an entire span of services, including treatment of any relevant withdrawal syndrome, lectures, group counseling, advice regarding jobs, and outreach to your family. In fact, the most important lessons offered are given in a repetitive way in order to maximize the chances that these lessons are learned and thought through thoroughly. Often, learning new ways of thinking about a change in lifestyle and developing abstinence require a bit of time to "mull things over." In light of today's financial realities, almost all inpatient rehabilitation programs attempt to teach these lessons of abstinence and life changes in two or three weeks or less. The staff of these programs know that what is learned will be relearned repeatedly during the aftercare phase.

In other words, within reason, the decision about the length of your inpatient program is hardly monumental. Indeed, it is likely that the "optimal" length of inpatient care will be dictated for you through all of the other considerations outlined here.

Other "Special" Considerations

One "special" consideration in choosing a program concerns the *characteristics of the other people receiving care*. Whereas much of the time spent in a program is structured, a significant portion of the day consists of talking with other people in treatment during breaks, over meals, and in the evenings. It is here that much of the "mulling over" and thinking things through occur. Therefore, it makes some sense that you consider the different styles of communication that people have. For example, some men and women prefer to be in programs with no mixing of the sexes, some prefer to affiliate with "blue-collar" men and women who tend to "speak the same language," and others seek out programs that tend to cater to people with professional degrees. Some people have a preference for a program with a strong religious component, whereas others want as little emphasis on God as possible. These are highly individual decisions, which are likely to have only a small impact on the actual outcome, but they are considerations that can affect the level of comfort you experience while going through rehabilitation.

A second special consideration is the *size of the program*. In the long run, this probably has little overall impact because even large treatment facilities tend to break people up into "treatment teams" or groups that are rarely larger than 15 patients. Nonetheless, some people might choose a larger program in the hope that this offers a greater cross section of patients, a larger staff with which to interact, and more recreational facilities. Others might choose smaller programs in the hope that the interactions that do occur will be a bit more individualized and personal.

An additional special consideration involves the *preferences* you might have developed *for a specific mode of therapy*. For example, some men and women with cocaine problems decide on their own that they want a specific type of medication to help them decrease craving. Similarly, many people addicted to heroin are certain that they want methadone treatment, although this therapy is only offered by a limited number of treatment facilities. Finally, some people with alcohol problems may be attracted to the more mechanical and behavioral approach offered by one chain of hospitals, which teaches them to become nauseated when they taste or smell their favorite alcoholic beverage. Obviously, if you have decided that you want to pursue a particular mode of therapy, this will be yet another consideration to bear in mind when selecting a treatment program appropriate to your needs.

In summary, as you will learn in the next chapter, inpatient (and outpatient) treatment programs are much more similar than they are different. It is also fairly clear that the choice of a particular program often rests with circumstances beyond your control (including your finances or the dictates of your insurer), or happenstance (including the experiences of your friends and family or the preferences of the person who helped you to confront your problems). Still, even though these issues are unlikely to have a major impact on whether you do well or poorly following the initial phases of rehabilitation, this chapter has shown that there are a variety of things to consider in selecting a program.

A Note to Family and Friends

Sometimes the crises involved with substances are so over-whelming, or the person involved with alcohol and drugs is so perplexed, that the selection of a particular program rests with family members and friends. Although this chapter has already given you all the information you require, there are a number of additional things you might consider.

First of all, you should recognize that whereas it is hard enough to make a choice that impacts on your own life, it is often even more frightening to take on the responsibility of such choices as they impact on someone else. This is even more difficult when the person is someone you know and love. Making matters still worse is the nagging feeling some of you may have about whether you are "really" deciding what's best for your relative or friend, or you are just trying to get rid of a difficult and frustrating situation.

Here, I can offer you some heartfelt reassurance. Remember that there are hundreds of potential combinations of appropriate therapies. There aren't any obvious "right" or "wrong" choices. The important thing is to give some sort of rehabilitation a chance to "take." Of much less importance is whether the program is inpatient or outpatient, large or small, situated in a rural or urban area, and so on. Just get help!

A final word of advice is in order. I have told you before and will repeat again an important lesson that is easily forgotten. Drug and alcohol problems are long-term difficulties, and they usually continue for long periods of time for reasons that none of us fully understands. We all agree that these factors relate to a person's inability either to admit to his or her problems or to acknowledge the relationship between life difficulties and sub-stance use, but the specific mechanism through which this occurs is unclear. Thus, intervention often involves a series of repeated efforts to teach the individual about the problems and to discuss the options he or she may have in getting rid of the difficulties. Similar statements can be made about rehabilitation. If the first inpatient or outpatient effort doesn't "take," this does not necessarily mean that the "wrong" program was selected. Rather, the drug or alcohol user often makes a series of slow steps forward after numerous efforts at intervention by family and friends. Sometimes, several efforts at rehabilitation are required before the user achieves an intense enough commitment to abstinence.

A Recap

So many pages, but such a straightforward message! This chapter was written to try to answer the questions many people face after they recognize that they have a serious substance problem and that something must be done about it.

There is a tendency that we all have to search and search for the "true" program. It is as if we believe that our only hope is in finding the one program that will save us. Well, as you will certainly learn in the next chapters, there is *nothing magical* to save us. Finding our way out of the program is a long-term process of relearning and rebuilding. With effort, treatment can be successful with inpatient or outpatient care, a large or small program, or in an urban or a rural setting. Lots of important considerations go into helping people to find the program they actually use. Most of these influences are common sense, happenstance, and financial considerations. Few (if any) are essential to recovery.

Additional Readings

Holder, H., and Blose, J. The reduction of health care costs associated with alcoholism treatment: A 14-year longitudinal study. *Journal of Studies on Alcohol* 53:293–302, 1992.

McLellan, A. Alcoholism: Treatment and outcomes. *Alcohol Digest* 41:11, 1994.

Schuckit, M. Treatment of alcoholism in office and outpatient settings. In: Mendelson, J. H., and Mello, N. K. (Eds.), *Medical Diagnosis and Treatment of Alcoholism*. New York: McGraw-Hill, 1992, pp. 363–392.

Walsh, D. C., Hingson, R. W., Merrigan, D. M., Levenson, S. M., Cupples, A., Heeren, T., Coffman, G. A., Becker, C. A., Barker, T. A., Hamilton, S. K., McGuire, T. G., and Kelly, C. A. Treatment options for alcohol abusing workers. *New England Journal of Medicine* 335:775–782, 1991.

8

What's Going on There?
A Guide to Detoxification

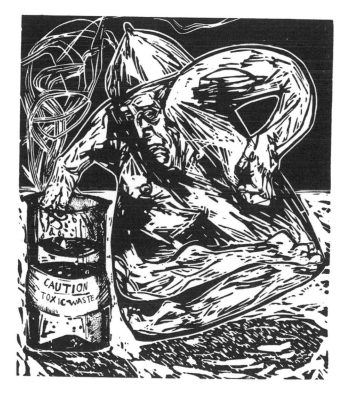

Figure 8.1 This figure illustrates a person trapped in a teapot in which he or she has steeped for months or years. The isolation and exposure to the chemicals in the container have caused the accumulation of harmful chemicals with subsequent toxic effects. Similarly, the process of detoxification, or ridding the body of the chemicals and promoting healing from their bruising consequences, is straightforward. Your body is already equipped to pour out the accumulated toxins. The process is rarely painful, often surprisingly simple, and this is an important first step in recovery.

Goals

When you really think about it, it is amazing that two fairly short chapters (Chapters 8 and 9) can be written to describe the general topic of "treatment programs." I am faced with the task of offering some thoughts that apply to inpatient and outpatient therapies, hospital-based and free-standing facilities, and to treatments that help people who are having problems with a wide variety of drugs. How is it possible to state general rules that apply to helping marijuana smokers, alcoholics, and people whose problems involve heroin or cocaine?

Actually, the task I face is no different from someone trying to give an overview of what an appendectomy is or what is likely to happen when you visit your dentist. What occurs in such settings, even in different cities or different parts of the world, follows a similar general pattern. It is only some of the details that differ.

Therefore, when a doctor or social worker considers how to help someone who walks into his or her office, he or she usually follows a fairly straightforward number of steps. These include evaluation, sharing the diagnosis (intervention), and helping someone choose a specific program. You have already learned a good deal about how these are accomplished. Once a setting for treatment is selected, then the health care professional has to consider whether formal detoxification (treatment for drug withdrawal) is required. A discussion of detoxification is what Chapter 8 is all about. Chapter 9 will then discuss what needs to be done in the initial stages of rehabilitation and beyond.

Is Detoxification Required?

This question at this stage of treatment focuses on whether physical addiction has occurred and, if so, the steps that can be followed in helping someone to go through the initial stages of withdrawal. As you learned in Chapter 2, while some mild symptoms like nervousness or headaches might be seen after stopping some drugs (including marijuana), the need for treatment of detoxification is only relevant to a few groups of drugs. Despite all of the other problems they cause, physical addiction to the point of requiring active treatment of withdrawal symptoms is *not* a problem associated with the marijuana-type drugs, hallucinogens, PCP, the solvents or inhalants, and so on. Difficulties with physical-withdrawal symptoms are *only* likely to be observed with the stimulants (including all forms of cocaine and amphetamine), the depressants (including alcohol, the Valium-type drugs, and the barbiturates), and the opiates (including heroin, codeine, and most of the prescription painkillers).

What Are the Symptoms of Withdrawal?

It is fairly easy to predict what withdrawal symptoms will look like, because they are usually the *opposite* of what the drug did the first time it was taken. This means that withdrawal from depressants such as alcohol is characterized by trouble sleeping, anxiety, a tremor of the hands, and increases in the heartbeat rate, blood pressure, and body temperature. Similarly, withdrawal from painkilling drugs such as codeine or heroin is characterized by pain in the muscles, bones, and joints, as well as by trouble sleeping, anxiety, diarrhea, and a runny nose. Finally, withdrawal from stimulant drugs such as amphetamines or cocaine is associated with fatigue, sleeping too much, an inability to concentrate, lack of self-confidence, and feelings of sadness.

There are some additional general guidelines that can help you understand what is likely to happen when you stop taking any member of these three classes of drugs. The first of these additional general issues relates to the time span over which you can expect to experience symptoms. The major factor involved here is understanding how long the drug had its effect each time you took it. The longer the initial actions of the drug, the longer the period of time that will pass before symptoms begin, and the longer the symptoms are likely to last. To use alcohol as an example, this is a drug that has a relatively short period of action (perhaps several hours). For alcohol and other drugs that produce an intoxication that lasts for several hours, symptoms of withdrawal (again, generally the opposite of the acute effects of that drug) are likely to begin within four to eight hours or so, reach peak intensity on approximately day two, and decrease fairly rapidly on days three, four, and five. A similar time frame for acute withdrawal is likely to be seen for other short-acting brain depressants such as Serax (oxazepam), Ativan (lorazepam), the shorter-acting forms of amphetamine, as well as all forms of cocaine, and for heroin.

The longer-acting drugs, those that produce intoxications that can last for many hours, are likely to produce a different time frame of withdrawal (if high enough doses of the drug have been taken over a long enough period of time). So, for example, people who have developed physical dependence on the relatively long-lasting Valium (diazepam) or Librium (chlordiazepoxide)—brain-depressant drugs of the benzodiazepine type—have a very different time course of withdrawal. These drugs, capable of producing effects for many hours and with some left-over effects likely to be seen a day or two after the initial intoxication, are associated with an onset of withdrawal symptoms that only begins several days after drug use has stopped or markedly diminished. Here, the time of peak intensity of withdrawal symptoms is not likely to be observed until perhaps five to seven days after the drug is decreased. Also, withdrawal symptoms are likely to last for two or three weeks, although, thankfully, at a decreasing intensity. A similar pattern of withdrawal symptoms is likely to be observed for other very long-acting drugs such as methadone.

In looking at the time course of withdrawal for physically addicting substances, it is important to remember a lesson briefly reviewed in Chapter 3. The acute or more intense withdrawal syndrome is over in a matter of days or weeks, but it is almost always followed by a longer term or protracted withdrawal that takes three to six months to disappear. Here, the same type of symptoms of insomnia, anxiety, depression, and changes in pulse rate that are seen during acute withdrawal are observed, but these persist at a much lower level of intensity. It does not appear that there is any difference in the length or intensity of the protracted withdrawal for shorter-acting or longer-acting drugs.

This section has emphasized information on what you can expect during acute and protracted withdrawal from depressant, stimulant, and opiate drugs. No other classes of drugs are likely to produce a severe withdrawal condition. Some doctors think that some mild problems like headache or nausea are occasionally seen after long-term use of marijuana or hallucinogens. However, it is not clear that those drugs really caused the symptoms. In any event, such discomfort is mild and is likely to last a few hours or days.

Finally, I recognize that I cannot give all the details about all types of substances. Nicotine dependence, for example, is a very important health problem. Whether consumed through smoking cigarettes, inhaling cigar or pipe smoke, or through snorting snuff or chewing tobacco, nicotine has major effects on the brain, many of which are similar to those of a mild stimulant drug. People do develop a physical dependence on nicotine, and this substance can be very hard to give up. So, several of the readings offered in the *References* relate to nicotine dependence and approaches that can be used in helping people to stop smoking. On the other hand, to keep this text readable and useful, I have focused most intensively on "the harder drugs," including alcohol.

How Are Withdrawal Symptoms Treated?

Some General Thoughts

Because most withdrawal states are relatively mild, treatment is usually simple. It involves offering good physical care, good nutrition and vitamins, and lots of reassurance that at least the worst part of the syndrome will be over within two to four days for most drugs. Because you or someone you care about might be facing treatment for alcohol or other drug withdrawal, I thought a brief review of what is likely to happen might be of interest.

The first step of treatment you are likely to encounter is a thorough physical exam. The goal is to identify and treat any medical problems that might have developed during the period of heavy use of alcohol or other drugs. Being in optimal physical shape is a good general goal for the treatment of any physical condition, and it is likely to make any withdrawal symptoms that might develop less intense.

Education, rest, and reassurance during withdrawal can also be remarkably helpful. It is extremely important that you learn as much as possible about the usual mild nature of the symptoms and the relatively short period of time over which discomfort is likely to be experienced.

In summary, withdrawal symptoms that are severe enough to interfere significantly with day-to-day functions are only seen following relatively high-intensity use of depressants, opiates, and stimulants. These withdrawal symptoms are almost always mild-to-moderate in intensity and rarely include severe life-threatening problems. The most noticeable symptoms are likely to be seen during the first several days for most shorter-acting drugs, and the prominent symptoms rarely last more than several weeks even for the longer-acting drugs such as Valium or methadone. The most important steps for a person in treatment involve recognizing the symptoms that are likely to occur and remembering that these problems are likely to be short-lived and are not likely to be intense.

Some forms of withdrawal, especially those related to brain depressants and opiates, can be partly alleviated by medications. These pharmacological treatments are very specific, meaning they are different for the different categories of drugs. The next section briefly reviews medications that can be appropriate for specific types of withdrawals.

Medications Likely to Be Used for Withdrawal from Depressants Like Alcohol

The Optimal Approach, Using Depressant Medications

 The purpose of this and the following section is *not* to teach people how to treat themselves during alcoholic or other brain-depressant withdrawal. The decisions regarding whether a medication makes any sense to use, as well as the optimal use of the nonmedicinal approaches, can only be made after relatively intense training and lots of clinical experience. However, consistent with all of the other information offered in this text, I believe that the more you understand about what you are going through, the easier things are likely to become. Therefore, the thoughts that are offered here help to increase your general knowledge of what medications might be chosen, and why.

In viewing specific medications, it is important to remind yourself why withdrawal symptoms are being observed in the first place. Your brain has become conditioned to having a brain depressant (alcohol, barbiturate, or a Valium-like drug) around. Because these substances are foreign to the body, the brain and other parts of the nervous system have built up defenses to resist the effects of these drugs, changes that took days to weeks to develop. Therefore, it makes sense that it takes days to weeks for the body to return to normal.

In large part, the symptoms of withdrawal are a result of the brain trying to cope with a fairly rapid change in its environment. After working to resist drug effects, all of a sudden the drugs are not available. Therefore, the essential step in pharmacological treatment of withdrawal, especially for brain depressants as well as for opiates, is to give the body brain depressants at adequate doses and then to take them away much more slowly. The slow disappearance of the depressant drugs from the body allows the nervous system time to adapt.

At least theoretically, any brain-depressant drug could be used to treat brain-depressant withdrawal. So, no matter which of the depressants a person has developed physical addiction to, symptoms are likely to be much less if any other brain depressant, or the drug of addiction, is readministered and slowly withdrawn. Thus, the alcohol withdrawal syndrome can be treated with alcohol, barbiturates, or Valium-like drugs; Valium withdrawal could be treated with barbiturates or Valium-like drugs; and so on.

In summary, brain-depressant withdrawal is often treated by administering some brain-depressant medication in high enough doses to cause a marked improvement in symptoms. Then, just by the passage of time, the brain and other parts of the nervous system are taught how to function normally in the absence of brain depressants by slowly decreasing the level of the brain depressant (such as Valium or Librium) that is used. When a short-acting drug has produced the physical dependence (for example, alcohol or Serax), the optimal amount of medication is given on day one, and the doses are decreased to zero by day four or five. When a long-acting brain depressant has produced physical dependence (as would be seen with physical addiction that had developed to Valium), the decrease in the level of the medication generally occurs over several weeks. When used in appropriate doses, these depressant drugs can markedly diminish the intensity of withdrawal symptoms. Most people only experience symptoms that resemble a mild flu.

Don't forget, however, that not everyone needs medications during depressant-withdrawal treatment. For some people, the symptoms are mild enough that education, reassurance, and general supports are sufficient.

Other Possible Approaches Using Medications

Because most withdrawal syndromes are relatively mild, it is possible just to treat specific symptoms like anxiety or a high pulse rate, rather than to use a medication that applies to the more global withdrawal syndrome. Therefore, although brain-depressant drugs are preferable, specific symptoms can be diminished with a variety of other medications. A blood pressure pill,

Catapres (clonidine), can help decrease some of the symptoms of high blood pressure and the fast pulse likely to be seen during withdrawal, can decrease any tremor of the hands, and can aid in sleeping. Another pill controlling blood pressure, Inderol (propranolol), can similarly help decrease symptoms. Of course, additional help can occur through the use of aspirin-like drugs for aches or pains, and so on.

Readings relevant to Chapter 8 discuss the potential usefulness of Catapres, and present information on another drug, chloromethiazole. However, most treatment programs use the brain depressants Valium, Librium, or Serax to treat alcohol withdrawal.

Medications for the Treatment of Opiate Withdrawal

The Use of Opiates

 The general rules offered regarding medicinal treatments for brain depressants apply here as well. With physical addiction to drugs like heroin or Demerol, withdrawal symptoms (most prominently the opposite of the acute effects of opiate drugs) have occurred because the brain and other parts of the nervous system have adapted to high levels of opiate drugs in the body. Therefore, the symptoms can improve a great deal if any opiate drug is given in a high enough dose on day one of withdrawal, and then the level of medication used is slowly decreased. Following addiction to the short-acting opiate heroin, the opiate used for treatment would be offered in the highest dose on day one, and the person would be weaned off of opiates by day four or five. For a physical dependence on longer-acting drugs (for example, methadone), it is likely to take two or three weeks or even longer of decreasing doses of an opiate to treat the withdrawal symptoms.

Almost any opiate can be used for the treatment of withdrawal. Therefore, people addicted to Darvon (propoxyphene) could be withdrawn with decreasing doses of Darvon, but they could also be treated with decreasing doses of another opiate, methadone. Also, at least theoretically, people addicted to codeine could be treated with Darvon, methadone, or almost any opiate in diminishing doses. However, in practice, most people physically addicted to opiates are withdrawn using decreasing doses of the specific opiate drug they are addicted to, or through the use of methadone. As described more fully in Chapter 9, methadone is a very powerful opiate itself, but it has the advantage of being relatively slowly destroyed by the body, and is well asorbed when taken by mouth. This means the drug can be taken once a day and that you don't have to be given shots. This makes it one of the easiest opiates to use for the treatment of withdrawal.

When adequate doses of opiates are used for the treatment of opiate withdrawal, the symptoms experienced by anyone going through this abstinence syndrome are likely to be fairly mild.

Other Possible Approaches Using Medications

As is true for any medication-based treatment, there are many variations and alternatives that can be considered. In fact, there are legal restrictions that *require* that some of these alternate approaches be used. Many states, including my own, California, do not allow the usual physician to prescribe opiate-type drugs for withdrawal to individuals known to be addicted to opiates. Under these circumstances, what can be done?

The good news is that the withdrawal from opiates, while capable of producing great discomfort, produces few, if any, life-threatening complications. It is not expected that anyone going through withdrawal will become terribly confused or develop convulsions as can be rarely seen during depressant withdrawal. In addition, most men and women who are taking opiate-type drugs such as heroin on the streets, are actually receiving relatively impure products that might only have 5% or 10% of heroin. Thus, withdrawal symptoms can be expected to be relatively mild for the average individual, and people are likely to respond well to education and reassurance that symptoms will be mild and short-lived.

The second bit of good news is that some of the most distressing symptoms of opiate withdrawal can be greatly improved through the use of nonopiate drugs. Although opiates would be preferable because they can decrease all of the symptoms, there are alternative approaches that can help. The type of pain in the muscles and bones likely to be experienced during withdrawal can be markedly improved by some of the nonopiate painkillers, including Tylenol (acetaminophen) and various forms of ibuprofen (such as Nuprin). The stuffy nose and coughs are often greatly improved by over-the-counter decongestants that are used to treat cold symptoms. Also, abdominal pain and symptoms of diarrhea are likely to be relieved by over-the-counter medications such as Kaopectate. In addition, the general agitation and flu-like feelings are likely to improve as part of the sleepiness caused by drugs such as Catapres (clonidine). In fact, because of the legal restrictions on the use of opiates for treating opiate withdrawal in California, most clinicians have found that a mixture of these various nonopiate medications aimed at specific symptoms, along with reassurance and education, can be very helpful.

Medications for the Treatment of Stimulant Withdrawal

Contrary to the prior two discussions of the treatment of depressant and opiate withdrawal, the description regarding stimulants can be handled fairly quickly. For a variety of reasons, careful studies have tended *not* to reveal any specific medication that is superior to the passage of time alone in dealing with stimulant withdrawal. Thankfully, many of the symptoms of withdrawal from stimulants can be relieved by eating frequent meals, by sleeping in response to the feelings of tiredness, and through reassurance that these symptoms are, indeed, quite temporary. Unfortunately, no medication appears to improve on this condition.

A number of studies have looked at the possibility of using a stimulant-type drug to treat stimulant withdrawal (1). Most of these investigations have looked at the relatively mild stimulant

Ritalin (methylphenidate). Despite the theory that stimulant drugs might help, there is little evidence that the withdrawal syndrome is at all improved by their use. Additional studies have looked at the possibility that other medications, especially those that alter the brain levels of the neurochemical dopamine, could also help withdrawal (2). Once again, when more carefully controlled studies are used, these dopamine-boosting drugs, such as Parlodel (bromocriptine), do not seem to offer any advantage over the passage of time and education along with re-assurance (1).

In summary, at the present time *no* medications are appropriate for treating people during stimulant withdrawal. Although studies have evaluated the use of stimulants, antidepressant drugs, and specific dopamine-boosting drugs, for none of these approaches do the assets appear to outweigh the financial costs and the side effects of the medications (1).

The one exception to these statements regarding medications for stimulant withdrawal applies to the drug nicotine. For many reasons, this product of tobacco is not a typical stimulant, and in my text aimed at professionals in the health care fields, nicotine and caffeine are described in a section by themselves. Nonetheless, it is probably useful to make brief mention here to some of the information offered on nicotine gum, such as Nicorette, and nicotine patches. The theory governing their use is that the symptoms of nicotine withdrawal could be improved by giving the individual a level of nicotine and then diminishing the dose over a period of time. Whether given as a type of chewing gum or applied to the skin through a bandaid-like patch, the weaning off nicotine does appear to be superior to the use of no medication at all for individuals who are not able otherwise to stop smoking. The tiredness, irritability, and increased appetite as well as other symptoms likely to be observed during withdrawal from this relatively weak stimulant do appear to improve when nicotine gum or nicotine patches are used. However, these approaches are only beneficial when used along with a formal smoking-cessation treatment approach that also educates people about nicotine and the withdrawal symptoms, motivates them to keep working toward abstinence, and teaches behaviors and attitudes that help them learn to live without the drug. The nictone product administration on its own does not appear to be sufficient.

Some Concluding Remarks

Obviously, a full and detailed description of withdrawal syndromes and their treatments cannot be handled here, although other sections of this book (particularly Chapters 3 and 6) give you additional information. The full story is best offered in medical texts. What is important is that stopping most drugs does not result in a withdrawal syndrome. Also, the treatment of withdrawal from even physically addicting drugs can be handled adequately with rest, education, and reassurance (as occurs, for example, for the stimulants). Most withdrawal syndromes require medications for only short periods of time. And whereas some withdrawal states, especially those associated with the brain depressants (for example, alcohol and the Valium-type drugs) can be severe, such intense states are definitely the exception and not the rule.

For the purposes of this text, it is important to say that many programs do not have a distinct detoxification component. Rather, the programs often combine detoxification with the inpatient or outpatient rehabilitation program. This can be done because most drugs have no withdrawal syndrome associated with them, and the three classes of agents that do involve withdrawal syndromes are likely to involve relatively mild symptoms. Even among these physically addicting drug classes, treatment sometimes involves no medications. In most circumstances, the medications that are used tend to be dropped by the end of the first week.

For most people, therefore, the recognition of a problem, selection of a program, and beginning of treatment leads directly into rehabilitation. Other people are more slowly introduced to rehabilitation during their first week of care as their physical withdrawal symptoms decrease. This transition from detox to rehab can occur either as an outpatient or an inpatient.

A Note to Family and Friends

I hope this chapter has helped you to understand more about what withdrawal symptoms are like and how they are optimally treated. The reason to review this information briefly is so that you have a greater understanding of what your loved one or friend is going through and of what options are available for helping him or her. Perhaps the most important way you can help someone going through withdrawal is to remind him that (although it often doesn't seem this way while he is actually experiencing symptoms) the discomfort associated with withdrawal is relatively short-lived and almost never life-threatening.

References

1. Schuckit, M. A. *Drug and Alcohol Abuse: A Clinical Guide to Diagnosis and Treatment,* Fourth Edition. New York: Plenum Medical Book Company, 1995.
2. Roehrich, H., Dackis, C., and Gold, M. Bromocriptine. *Medical Research Reviews* 7:243–269, 1987.

Additional Readings

Chang, G., and Koster, T. R. Detoxification. In Lowinson, J. H., Ruiz, P., Milliman, R. B., and Langrod, J. G. (Eds.), *Substance Abuse: A Comprehensive Textbook,* Third Edition. Baltimore: Williams & Wilkins, 1997, pp. 377–382.

Kenof, P. D., Aronson, M. J., and Ness, R. Organic mood syndrome associated with detoxification from methadone maintenance. *American Journal of Psychiatry* 150:423–428, 1993.

Meyer, R. New pharmacotherapies for cocaine dependence. *Archives of General Psychiatry* 49:900–904, 1992.

Satel, S. L., Kosten, T. R., Schuckit, M. A., and Fischman, M. W. Should protracted withdrawal from drugs be included in DSM-IV. *American Journal of Psychiatry* 150:695–704, 1993.

9

What's Going on There? A Guide to Rehabilitation

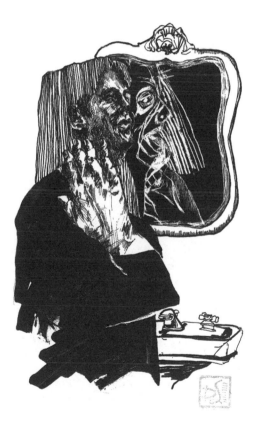

Figure 9.1. Standing on the outside of a treatment program and looking in can be very frightening. In some ways, the feelings can resemble what goes through your mind when you pass by a mirror and hardly recognize the reflection facing you. You are likely to have fears regarding what you are about to go through, especially in light of concerns that you might be having about your own abilities. However, as demonstrated in this illustration, even if the reflection appears distorted, much of what you are seeing is likely to be the result of alcohol and drugs and not the real you. You are likely to be amazed both at how strong your abilities remain and at the manner in which the rehabilitation process helps you once again to get in touch with the real you.

What Really Is "Rehabilitation"?

No matter who you are, what drug is involved, or the circumstances of your life, rehabilitation for a substance use disorder is fairly straightforward. It involves helping to be sure you are as physically healthy as possible, helping you to recognize how important abstinence from substance use is to you, and offering you advice and support as you begin to rebuild your life without alcohol or drugs. This last process includes an approach called **relapse prevention** that will help you to stay clean and sober even after the more intense phase of treatment is done.

The First Goal: Increasing Your Level of Physical and Psychological Functioning

The need to make sure you are as healthy as possible is a matter of simple common sense. After all, if stopping substance use is difficult, detoxification has its own stresses, and rebuilding a life without alcohol or drugs requires effort and concentration. It is extremely difficult to accomplish all these steps if you are physically impaired or confused. Therefore, all treatment programs begin with a good physical evaluation.

For most people who have had problems with alcohol or drugs, the need to identify and treat medical problems is obvious. No matter how young or resilient you are, heavy doses of alcohol or drugs can inflame the liver, cause problems with other body organs such as the heart, lungs, and pancreas, and leave you open to all sorts of infections. Thus, an important first step in any rehabilitation effort is a thorough medical examination to identify and correct any treatable physical problems. An important related step is allowing for the passage of time so that the body can heal, as it almost certainly will with abstinence.

Substance-related problems with thinking are frequently referred to as being "wet." This means that, just as the liver and stomach develop problems as they try to protect themselves from the onslaught of alcohol and drugs, so, too, the brain becomes a bit battered and bruised. What is probably involved in this damage is a series of changes in salts, sugars, cell membrane components, and other brain chemicals that impair the ability of the brain to regulate moods and think clearly. With rest and good nutrition, and in the absence of any obvious evidence of major damage that should be identifiable by your physician, your ability to concentrate, think things through carefully, and to control mood swings is likely to be appreciably improved within several days to several weeks of abstinence. Obviously these changes are important if you are to learn all that needs to be learned during treatment. Here, it is the passage of time that makes the difference—medications or psychotherapies might not have a major impact at this point.

Because many people with substance use disorders do develop temporary problems with brain functioning, they may at first find it difficult to understand and remember the lessons they are taught during the early stages of rehabilitation. As a result, most formal treatment programs tend to teach the same major lessons several times before the end of the more intensive rehabilitation phase. The fact that different patients have different levels of temporary problems with brain functioning also makes it difficult to develop a hard-and-fast rule about how long the initial phase of rehabilitation should continue. In any event, all the treatment programs I know of recognize the need to *optimize functioning*. Although they might not officially highlight this step in their brochures, it remains an important focus of almost all early treatment efforts.

The Second Goal: Becoming Motivated to Stop Using Alcohol and Drugs (and to Stay Stopped)

This section begins to describe issues likely to be covered during group sections and educational lectures. Some of these important topics are listed in Table 9.1.

Table 9.1
Topics Often Discussed in Substance-Related Rehabilitation Programs

- The nature or characteristics of dependence
- The problems caused by substances
- The need to abstain from all substances of abuse
- Discussions of how other people have recovered
- The importance of self-help groups like AA, NA, and CA
- The roles family members and friends can serve in rehabilitation
- The use of free time when sober
- How to rebuild personal relationships
- How to handle social situations where alcohol and drugs are available
- The need to avoid "using" friends
- Having fun when "clean"

Why Abstinence?

The very wording of this subheading raises a question. It is easy to understand why motivation is important, but it is not always so clear to everyone why this has to include abstinence. It is also unclear to many people why abstinence is usually meant to include *all* substances, not just the major drug that might have precipitated the need for treatment.

People with substance difficulties are usually able to stop use temporarily. Most people seem to abstain time after time when a social crisis or physical problem develops. Unfortunately, their ability to clean up or dry out often convinces them that they do not have a problem with the substance.

The usual (I would almost say *universal*) course of problems with alcohol or drugs also involves periods of time when the pattern of substance use shows temporary evidence of control. Therefore, the alcoholic *can* go to a party and have only two drinks, *can* restrict himself or herself to only one type of beverage (like beer) taken at a particular time of day, and *can* limit the number of days of the week on which drinking occurs. In a similar manner, the person having problems with marijuana, codeine, and even stimulants can often limit his or her intake of the substance to certain times or certain situations. So, control (at least for a period of time) is not the central issue here.

The real issue is consistency of control. Almost by definition, the fact that someone has identified a serious enough difficulty to consider treatment, and then seek help, indicates that *every time* in the past that abstinence was achieved and rules of control were followed, eventually intake escalated, and further problems developed. Because the pattern of past behaviors is a very good predictor of future behavior, it is obvious that any use in the future is eventually going to lead to escalation of intake and associated problems.

There are excellent studies that demonstrate that this "off and on again" nature of substance-related problems is the rule rather than the exception. Although most of the investigations were carried out by those studying alcohol, the results apply to other drugs as well (1, 2). To my knowledge, every study that has followed groups of alcoholics over time has not only documented the tendency for repeated periods of temporary abstinence and controlled patterns of use, but has shown that among those with difficulties severe enough to be diagnosed as alcoholism, the resumption of use almost always leads to future problems (1, 3). This may take days, weeks, or even months to develop, but the difficulties *will* occur.

Therefore, if the goal of rehabilitation is to decrease the chances of further problems to as close to zero as possible, the process must include abstinence. This statement does not come from any emotional preference on my part. It is just the way things are. There is nothing that you or I can do to change the facts!

Why Abstinence from All Drugs?

By now, you might have reached a point where you can accept that abstinence from the drug that has caused you problems is an important part of treatment. But you still might be wondering why all other substances must be avoided. Believe me, if I could save you the pain and problems associated with avoiding all forms of alcohol and drugs, I would. Unfortunately, both common sense and evidence from scientific studies tell us that to maximize the chance of recovery, the use of all substances must stop. Maintaining abstinence and rebuilding a life without substances is so important and time-consuming that anything that decreases self-control or increases craving for substances is a severe threat to recovery. Alcohol and all drugs of abuse go to the brain, change how you feel, and almost always result in some sort of a floating sensation that often involves a feeling of freedom or lack of restrictions. You tend to forget problems and pain, feel that everything is rosy, and that the future will turn out to be wonderful, no matter what you do. This means that when you get high with any drug, even ones you don't have dependence on, your motivation for abstinence from the substance that has caused the most problems is likely to decrease. It's fairly easy to figure out what is likely to happen next.

Another reason to avoid all substances is that few people take one drug at a time. It is likely, for example, that you mixed a high from alcohol with one from marijuana and vice versa, that you used stimulant drugs to try to get going in the morning after you had been "high" from depressants such as alcohol or the Valium-type drugs, or that you turned to more sedating substances such as marijuana or the brain depressants to help come down from cocaine. Unfortunately, anything you associate in your mind with taking a substance is likely to increase your craving for it. Thus, just as the smell or taste of a drink of alcohol is likely to increase your desire for marijuana, the sedation you might feel with Valium-type drugs might increase your craving for stimulants.

Actually, I have just given an example of the types of things that treatment programs teach to help a person maximize and maintain the desire for abstinence. Some of the thoughts outlined here are likely to be offered during a rehabilitation program as part of a series of educational lectures, movies and videotapes, and during group counseling sessions.

How Does "Group Therapy" Help with Motivation?

Some of you might feel your heart skip a beat at the thought of "group therapy." Really, what goes on is very straightforward. It involves listening to other people who are wrestling with problems that are amazingly similar to yours and sharing some of your own fears and future plans with the group leaders and members. The emphasis is almost always on the here and now. The discussions review the personal prices paid in the past for substance use, offer appropriate plans for handling craving and situations where you find yourself "falling into" use of alcohol or drugs, and help you build a plan for how to keep your spirits and motivation high in the future. Few programs would "make you" talk about highly personal aspects of your life, and few focus on issues relating to how you grew up. The philosophy in most programs recognizes that there is a problem *now*—the question is what can be done about it.

In addition to lectures, movies, or videotapes, group discussions focus on present life circumstances. Almost all programs try to use the experiences of other people to show you that abstinence can be achieved and maintained. Much of this learning comes through interactions with counselors and teachers, some of whom are themselves recovering from similar problems. These activities help you to remember why abstinence is such an important part of building a new life and demonstrate that other people can make it—and so can you.

Other help in motivation occurs through self-help groups. The "grandaddy" of these groups, which have become an essential component of most treatment programs, is Alcoholics Anonymous.

Do I "Have to" Join a Self-Help Group?

I realize that no single text like this can hope to explain all of the details of AA, CA, NA, PA, Rational Recovery, and other important self-help groups. When you enter an inpatient or outpatient rehabilitation program, these groups will be explained, and you will have lots of chances to read and discuss issues about them. At this point, however, it is worth examining some misconceptions you might have about these groups.

First, although some people feel that it is possible to recover without a self-help group, there is no compelling reason to try to do so. All of these groups cost nothing, they are available twenty-four hours a day, and they are made up of people who sincerely want to help.

Second, there is no "cookbook" formula that all groups follow in exactly the same manner (4). However, these groups are likely to share some basic components. They all emphasize abstinence. All demand that you at least consider the obvious statement that you have lost control of your use of the substance (and subsequently lost control of many aspects of your life). All encourage you to work with people who have had similar experiences, and each is based on the premise that by sharing your experiences you will help yourself and others improve their lives. Many groups have adopted AA's twelve-step recovery program, a formula that, if followed fully, will not only lead to continued abstinence but also will help you to rebuild your life.

Although all of these statements are true, there are still huge differences between the various self-help groups. For example, some groups insist on an adherence to religious principles, but many do not. Some preach an unswerving acceptance of the twelve recovery steps, whereas others encourage people to view those steps as a guideline to be modified when needed. Some groups advise you to attend meetings almost nightly for a period of time, whereas others insist that attending several meetings per week is sufficient. Finally, some groups insist on a lifelong adherence to group participation, whereas others offer much more flexibility, advising you to use the group intensely for a number of months and then reevaluate how often you need to participate.

Any way you look at it, however, participation in a relevant self-help group helps to maximize the motivation for abstinence, and also helps contribute to rebuilding a life free of substances.

Every group I know of incorporates education, learning from others, the appropriate use of recovering men and women as a model for your own individualized recovery plans, and addresses most of the other steps outlined in this chapter. Indeed, many men and women achieve and maintain sobriety solely with the help of good general medical care and strong adherence to a self-help group. Many others opt to maximize their chances for recovery by incorporating every possible component, including more formal inpatient and outpatient rehabilitation.

Why Must My Family and Friends Be Involved?

Just as substance abuse affects everyone within reach of the person with problems, going through rehabilitation is not a solitary process.

Family members and friends rarely understand what went into the development of substance-related problems, how difficult it is to stop using despite the best intentions, and the complex series of steps involved in the hard work required for recovery. The more those around you learn about these issues, the more they will be able to understand what you are going through and offer support. Therefore, almost all treatment programs have groups where family members and friends can learn about what goes on during rehabilitation from alcohol and other substances. Many programs also incorporate joint counseling sessions that involve both friends and family members along with the person with substance problems.

The Third Goal: Rebuilding a Lifestyle Free of Substances

Whether you enter an inpatient or outpatient rehabilitation program, the lectures, tapes, self-help group meetings, and outreach to family and friends all have a second important agenda. The goal here is to help you and those around you recognize that substances have become such an important part of your life that giving them up can be difficult and painful. With this in mind, the educational meetings and group discussions introduce you to a series of problems you are likely to face when rebuilding your life without substances, including difficulties you might not have considered on your own. The goal is to *begin* a dialogue that is to be continued as you go out into the real world and attempt to apply what you have learned. Since these problems cannot be conquered overnight, this dialogue must continue for many months as part of aftercare.

The types of problems you are likely to face and that are the focus of this aspect of treatment include the following:

1. *What are you going to do with your free time?* Sounds simple, doesn't it? But if you really stop to think about it, a great deal of your time before or after work or school and on the weekends was spent preparing to take substances, actually ingesting them, and staying high or recovering from the effects of alcohol and drugs. Giving up all of those steps means that you have to learn how to fill your days, have fun, and establish and maintain relationships in a sober state. This requires planning, trial and error, and a willingness to bounce ideas off those around you.

2. *How are you going to relate to people when you are sober?* Most people would love to believe that, once they have made the decision to stop drinking or taking drugs, the world will be grateful. Unfortunately, things are a bit more complicated.

What is more likely to happen is that some people around you begin to realize how furious they really are. The problem is that while you were involved with alcohol and drugs, your sober friends and relatives were so concerned that you might crash your car, drop out of school or lose your job, or not come home (or come home stoned or drunk) that they rarely had the chance to get in touch with their own feelings about the situation. They are likely to have stopped up their anger, fears, and frustrations. Sure, some explosions of anger occurred, but these accomplished little and were often followed by feelings of guilt and even higher levels of frustration.

Now you return to your spouse, children, parents, and friends and say: "I'm back—love me!" The first reaction is likely to be one of relief on their part. However, this is often followed by accusations (both verbal and in more subtle forms) of "How could you have done that to me?" or "I know it's unfair, but I'm gonna make you pay." Anyone would have trouble handling anger and frustrations that have been built up over a period of many years. The thought of facing these stresses while you're still "wet" and dealing with your own problems can appear overwhelming.

That is one of the reasons why the educational lectures, group counseling, couples and family counseling, and all of the other steps inherent in rehabilitation are there for you. That is also why the more intense initial outpatient and inpatient phases of rehabilitation are only the beginning of working through these problems. Reestablishing relationships, or learning enough to be able to avoid similar mistakes in new relationships, is possible. In fact, these steps have been accomplished by millions of people. On the other hand, this takes time and is very difficult to do on your own. Thus, building and repairing relationships is an important part of what goes on during the rehabilitation process.

3. *How are you going to learn to say "no" when many of the situations and the people around you are pushing you to say "yes"?* Once intense and persistent substance use is in place, there are a host of factors that tend to keep the process going. These include swapping your old friends who are "clean" for a new peer group that is every bit as involved with substances as you are. Unfortunately, if you now spend time with your "using" friends after you've made a commitment to abstinence, it is not only likely that they will offer you alcohol or drugs, but they are likely to do everything possible to convince you to use them. After all, if they were as heavily involved with substances as you, and if they believe that they have no problem themselves, then they must believe that you do not have a problem. If you have a problem, so do they, and they are not willing to admit that.

Thus, part of group counseling, and the self-help groups, is to help you understand some of these issues and give you some options for developing clean and sober friends. When you stay around users, it is almost impossible to say "no," at least in the long run. Many programs also use lectures and group discussions to try to help you rehearse how you might assert your need for abstinence when offered alcohol or drugs. There are many tricks to be used in social situations and many ways to learn how to avoid environments where you are likely to use. Most of these steps are not obvious and require a learning process that is offered in all good rehabilitation programs.

Another important step in learning to say no involves considering the possibility that you might need changes in the specific structure of your job. For example, how will you handle yourself if you're invited to "go out with the guys" (or "girls") over lunch or after work? What will you do to occupy the time at night in a hotel room if you have to travel for a living? Therefore, many group discussions will deal with options that might be available to you. Many programs often have educational and vocational counselors to work with you.

4. *How can you relax or feel comfortable without your drug?* You probably realized even before reading the material presented above that becoming comfortable with a new style of life requires the passage of time. The farther away you are from substance use, and the more time and effort that you have invested in developing a lifestyle free of substances, the easier it becomes to stay sober. As time goes on you are likely to discover that you can go to parties, interact with other people, and carry out all the other daily activities that are part of the world and enjoy yourself even though you are not high. However, what are you going to do until time passes?

Most programs recognize that additional efforts are needed here. Many facilities utilize group therapy and individual sessions to help you explore ways to function better. They then offer you the opportunity to exercise, increase your participation in religion if you wish, develop hobbies, and so on. Some programs also give more formal education about relaxation. These can include things such as meditation, biofeedback, and self-hypnosis. As fancy as the last sounds, it really only involves learning how to sit quietly, relax your muscles, and focus on pleasant and pleasing situations.

The Fourth Goal: Staying Clean and Sober or Relapse Prevention

This important step in learning how to recover and stay clean and sober is actually just a restatement of many of the important issues discussed in this chapter. Developed through a variety of theoretical approaches, each form of relapse prevention trains people to recognize situations that markedly increase the risk of returning to alcohol and drugs, teaches ways to avoid these high-risk situations, and focuses on the appropriate way to handle "a slip" if it does occur.

High-risk situations are any conditions where the physical surroundings and/or mood make a return to substance use a next natural step. Finding yourself calling "old friends" with whom you have used substances in the past and driving through old neighborhoods or stopping at bars that you used to frequent might appear to be chance or "apparently irrelevant" decisions, but they often are part of a barely conscious drive to get back to alcohol and drug use. Obviously the more time spent with users and the greater the proportion of the week you find yourself in situations where substances are easily available, the greater the likelihood that you will return to using.

Other high-risk situations involve mood states that either remind you of the "high" or bring back many of the feelings that occurred as complications of substance use, including withdrawal. Therefore, times when you are very tired, frustrated, angry, or feeling physically ill are periods of very high risk for many substance-dependent men and women. It is these feelings (just like old faces and old neighborhoods) that often have associated with them a reflex of reaching for the white powder, needle, or glass.

At the same time, people are human, and it is not always possible to control moods or situations. Therefore, a relapse-prevention program teaches you how to rehearse the "next step" when you find yourself in a high-risk situation. It is best to have planned out long ahead of time how to get out of the neighborhood, cope with the bad mood, or deal with the life hassles. Once you are in the uncomfortable situation and your craving for substance use has climbed, it is much more difficult to decide what to do. Rehearsing protective moves in a relapse-prevention group is often done in writing and/or verbally in front of others in the group. It is always important to see how other people have handled such situations successfully in the past.

Another cornerstone of any relapse prevention approach is the recognition that a temporary return to substance use *can* occur. At the same time that people are helping you to try to learn how to avoid such slips, there are a number of approaches that can be used to make sure that if one occurs, the period of substance use is as short as possible. One important component of relapse prevention is to recognize that there is no magical clock that only records *continuous* sobriety. So, it is not as if you are a downhill skier who fell on your effort to make record time, thus ruining your record bid. Here, it is the amount of sobriety and freedom from drugs overall that is important. Thus, a slip is not a disaster where you "lost" your days or months of sobriety. It is not an excuse to continue use, but it is an important lesson to be filed away as you dust yourself off and return to your program of recovery.

A Mini Recap

There are no magic cures for substance-related problems. Nor is it likely that anyone will be able to "make you recover."

It took many years for substance-related difficulties to develop. Alcohol and/or drugs have probably become a very important part of your life, and the process of recovery entails a lot of hard work on your part. It should not be surprising, therefore, that all rehabilitation programs just offer commonsense general help. The same types of approaches are used in inpatient and outpatient settings and can be applied to almost any type of substance-related difficulties. The treatment steps involve optimizing levels of physical and mental functioning, a series of efforts to help you to develop and maintain the highest possible level of motivation for abstinence, and a long-term ongoing effort to help you rebuild your life without alcohol and drugs. The process focuses on the here-and-now, does not dig deeply into your soul or psyche, and gives you nothing of which to be afraid. The steps are straightforward.

Additional Possible Treatment Components

Although almost every program incorporates almost all of the factors just outlined, there are several other possible approaches you might hear about. These include the potential role of medications and some behavioral approaches in the treatment of substance problems. These additional treatment components are briefly discussed below.

Medications

Some medications, such as those used for liver disease, are, of course, appropriately used to treat physical problems caused by substance use. Other medications can be used to treat the withdrawal syndrome from brain depressants or from opiates. However, few programs routinely use other medications for their patients. It is important for you to remember, however, that when an independent major psychiatric disorder occurs—such as manic depressive disease, schizophrenia, or severe and persisting depressions lasting beyond four to six weeks of abstinence—medications for the psychiatric conditions can be extremely important. Nonetheless, the majority of alcohol- and drug-dependent people do not have these conditions and, therefore, with some exceptions, the role of medications in most rehabilitation programs is relatively minor.

Medications Considered in the Treatment of Alcoholism

As discussed earlier, alcohol withdrawal can be effectively treated through the use of the Valium-type drugs for three to five days following abstinence. Once this period has ended, however, these benzodiazepine drugs have no place in the routine treatment of alcoholics. This is true even though continued sleeping problems and feelings of anxiety might persist for several months. The difficulty with the Valium-type drugs when taken on a daily basis is that they only remain clinically useful for anxiety or sleep problems for at most several weeks. As the medications lose effectiveness, the average person is tempted to increase the dose, which can in turn increase the risk for intoxication and problems with the prescribed drugs. So, it is rarely appropriate to use these benzodiazepines after detoxification has been completed.

Historically, many alcohol treatment programs have used a medication that alters the way in which the body breaks down or metabolizes alcohol. After taking Antabuse (disulfiram), usually in doses of about 250 milligrams a day, drinking alcohol can cause a serious reaction that induces nausea, vomiting, and rapid changes in blood pressure. Therefore, Antabuse is prescribed after detoxification is completed in the hope that the alcoholic cannot go back to drinking on the spur-of-the-moment. The drug is often used during aftercare for several months to perhaps a year following the end of the formal, intensive portion of the rehabilitation program. However, there is much debate about the effectiveness of this drug. Thus, there are no hard-and-fast rules about whether it is appropriate or inappropriate to use Antabuse during alcoholic rehabilitation. It is a drug worth considering, but it is not an essential part of care.

Many treatment programs are concerned about the high level of mood swings that are likely to be seen for several months following abstinence from alcohol. Most of the data from good studies tend to indicate that these mood swings are part of the body's readjustment to an existence without alcohol and do not represent a severe independent depressive disorder. On the other hand, it is important to remember that an accurate diagnosis of manic depressive disease indicates the need for lithium in anyone (including alcoholics and drug abusers), and that severe depressions lasting all day every day for many months in the absence of dependence on alcohol and drugs also indicate the need for *antidepressant* medications such as Pamelor (nortriptyline). However, these drugs have no place in the treatment of the usual alcoholic. The antidepressant drugs do not cause a stabilization in mood in the usual alcohol-dependent man or woman and do not increase the chances for abstinence.

Several other medications might hold some promise, in the future, in the treatment of alcoholism. Perhaps the most promising of these drugs is actually a medication that antagonizes or blocks the brain's ability to react to opiates like heroin. Trexan (naltrexone) is used in the treatment of heroin or other opiate overdoses, and it has some place in the treatment of the rehabilitation of opiate addicts. More information on this interesting approach as it applies to alcoholism is given in the *References*. Its use in the treatment for heroin addiction is described later in this chapter, although the effectiveness of this approach for heroin addicts does not appear to be very high. Recently, several studies have described the use of Trexan for alcoholics (5, 6). Although this drug has little effect on whether an alcohol-dependent man or woman will return to drinking after rehabilitation, those who take Trexan appeared to stop their alcohol use (go back on the wagon) much more rapidly than comparable individuals who were taking a placebo. Of course, Trexan is only of any potential importance if combined with all of the major aspects of the treatment programs described in this chapter. Even though the scientists investigating this drug don't understand why it might be helpful in alcoholism, they hypothesize that Trexan interferes with the "high" or intoxication received from alcohol. Because only two modest-sized studies have been published, I do *not* recommend that Trexan be routinely included in alcohol rehabilitation. However, I am watching further developments regarding this drug with great interest, and I might change my mind regarding the routine use of Trexan once more data are available.

There are several additional medications under investigation for the treatment of alcoholism. However, most treatment programs do not use them at present, and *I would not recommend that they be taken by anyone as part of alcohol rehabilitation until more data become available.* These potentially interesting drugs include an antianxiety medication called Buspar (buspirone), which is quite different from the Valium-type drugs. One of the readings gives a bit more detail. It is also possible that future studies will demonstrate that some drugs that affect the brain's level of the neurochemical serotonin might prove to be of some use in helping to decrease craving or diminish the effects of alcohol.

A very recent study in Europe has also raised the possibility that another drug, acamprosate, might produce the same type of results in alcoholics as does Trexan. Here too, more work will have to be done before this drug can be recommended for routine use.

Finally, one group of medications is described in the *References*. For thousands of years people have sought substances that will allow them to consume very high doses of alcohol but experience little or no effects. Named after a beautiful young woman in Greek mythology, these amythestic, or sobering, agents have been the subject of much speculation. However, good scientific studies have not yet revealed any specific drug that will allow people to enjoy the taste of alcohol but protect them from intoxication. Although caffeine does help counteract a few of the feelings of very *mild* intoxication, this is of no practical importance for even modest levels of drinking. Similarly, there are other approaches that can help speed up the rate of metabolism or breakdown of alcohol by perhaps 10% or 20%, but to date these substances have carried relatively high levels of side effects and subsequent dangers.

Medications Considered for Treating Problems with Stimulants (Cocaine and Amphetamine)

 This section is relatively easy to write since most rehabilitation programs aimed at people who have problems with stimulant drugs do not use any medications. However, for your general information, it is probably worthwhile to mention three types of pharmacological treatments that are *sometimes* considered for stimulant abusers but that should not be used on a routine basis until more studies have been done.

Probably the most commonly discussed agent is an antidepressant, usually Norpramin (desipramine) or Tofranil (imipramine). The theory is that the mood swings and craving that can be so intense after using any physically addicting drug, including the stimulants, might be improved by these drugs. This could be related to the general ability of antidepressant medications to help decrease mood swings, or might reflect a specific chemical change in the brain resulting from the use of the stimulant. In any event, there are several studies that reported that these antidepressant medications look promising (7). Unfortunately, there are as many investigations that cast doubt on their usefulness for stimulant rehabilitation. Because these medications cost money, and reflecting the dangers likely to occur if the antidepressants are mixed with cocaine or amphetamines, most programs do not routinely use these drugs as part of the rehabilitation efforts for stimulant dependence.

The second category of medications discussed for stimulant rehabilitation is an unusual agent that has its major effect on the brain chemical dopamine. Parlodel (bromocriptine) is usually used in medicine because of its ability to change dopamine in a way that stops women from producing milk after the birth of a baby. It is also useful for the treatment of some of the complications of certain brain tumors. As regards substance-related problems, however, it may prove useful in treatment because many of the stimulants have a major effect on that same brain chemical, dopamine. Therefore, it is possible that some of the symptoms seen during and after stimulant withdrawal, such as craving, *might* be helped with Parlodel. However, there are few convincing data from well-done studies, and it is not appropriate to prescribe this drug routinely at the present time.

Finally, the newest drug thought to be of possible help with readjustment to life after abuse of stimulants is Buprenex (buprenorphene). This is actually a painkiller, but it appears to have some unique effects in the brain and might impact on the desire to use stimulants. The data from the studies to this point, however, are very scanty (although promising). Because this drug is itself physically addicting and might even be sought out by substance abusers, it is best to be very careful before routinely using this agent. At the present time it should not be offered in the usual treatment program.

Medications for Treating Opiate Dependence

Physical addiction to codeine, heroin, the prescription painkillers, or methadone is followed by a physical withdrawal syndrome. Most physicians choose to treat these symptoms either with opiates (if the treatment program has a special license), or through the use of other medications that can help relieve symptoms (as described in Chapter 8).

Once detoxification has been completed, there are several possible pharmacological approaches for helping with opiate rehabilitation. There is not enough space to discuss them in detail here, but a brief mention is worthwhile.

First, it is possible that people who cannot otherwise become free of opiate drugs might do better taking an addicting agent that can be administered orally and only once a day. This agent is methadone or Dolophine, and its use is described further in the *References*. However, there are both pros and cons to methadone maintenance. Ideally, methadone is given in an attempt to help people to be able to go to work despite their opiate addiction and in the hope that, while taking this drug, they will not feel a need to use street heroin. It is important to remember that methadone must be used as part of a more comprehensive treatment program offering all the steps to increase motivation and to rebuild a life without drugs. If methadone decreases the use of street drugs IV, the risk for AIDS and other complications can be diminished. Although not a total success, the data do indicate that methadone can be useful in treating people with very severe opiate problems who do not respond to any other form of treatment (8). Ideally, methadone should be used for a year or so, and the person then should be gradually weaned off the substance. Unfortunately, getting people to stop taking methadone can be extremely difficult, and some individuals stay on this drug for a very long time.

Another interesting group of drugs has proven to be highly successful in the laboratory but a relative "bust" in the clinic. These agents, including naltrexone (Trexan), are medications that can block or antagonize the ability of other opiates to produce a high. However, despite all of the good things that can be said about Trexan, and regardless of its possible importance in the treatment of alcoholism, most opiate-dependent people who try this approach soon stop using the drug, often in a matter of days to weeks. Therefore, although some treatment programs aimed at helping people addicted to opiates offer these medications, and whereas I myself sometimes recommend them, it does not appear as if opiate antagonists are likely to work for most people.

Aversive Conditioning

At this point, it is important to remind you that the usual treatment program uses a combination of multiple approaches for rehabilitation and only very rarely resorts to medication and aversive conditioning. Therefore, when you are wondering what you are likely to face when you enter rehabilitation, pay attention to this entire chapter. If I had my druthers, because the treatments outlined in this subsection are less often used, I would recommend that you skip this section. On the other hand, you might be considering a program that offers medications or the form of behavior modification described here. In that case, these topics could be important to you.

There are many forms of behavior modification. I believe that all rehabilitation programs make some efforts at modifying behaviors through offering reassurance, and teaching ways to increase feelings of relaxation. So, the specific topic covered here is only one of many forms of efforts to modify behaviors **(behavior modification)**, just as there are many medications and many types of counseling approaches.

The concept of the specific behavioral treatment, **aversive conditioning,** is demonstrated by a personal experience I had. When I was a child, one night I ate lamb chops for dinner. Totally unrelated to that meal, later that evening I developed a severe case of the flu. As a result, I threw up lamb chops for hours. Lamb has a very specific taste, and my body automatically began to assume that it was the lamb that made me sick. Therefore, for years I could not stand the taste or smell of lamb in any form; it made me feel violently sick.

This natural process is a powerful example of aversive conditioning. As used in some treatment programs for alcoholism, people are given a drug that causes them to feel nauseated. As soon as they start to look "sick," they are asked to smell and taste their favorite alcoholic beverage. Then they throw up. After perhaps three to five treatments, even the sight or smell of that particular type of alcohol is likely to be met with nausea and even vomiting. These unpleasant feelings can be a useful reminder to the otherwise highly motivated person that drinking is bad for him or her.

On the other hand, 99% of treatment programs in the United States do not use this approach primarily because the requirement for nurses and physicians to administer the approach can be costly. It is difficult to be certain if this treatment component actually increases the recovery rate. However, since aversive conditioning has a long history, I felt it was important to mention it here.

What Are My Chances of Succeeding?

There are several reasons why the answer to this question is quite encouraging. First, a significant proportion of alcohol- and drug-dependent men and women, perhaps as many as 30%, go through what is called a permanent spontaneous remission (1). For reasons that no one really understands, they wake up one morning and say (for the hundredth time), "I've got to stop." And, again for the hundredth time, they do stop. The difference is that this time the cessation of intake of alcohol and drugs is permanent. Therefore, both those readers who are concerned about their own future as well as that of their family members and friends should always remember that the condition of alcohol or drug dependence is not hopeless. It is hard to predict when it will occur, but many people with severe alcohol and drug problems do permanently stop using without any formal treatment.

The second encouraging news is the relatively high rate of good outcomes among those people who are motivated to participate in care. These data relate to individuals who enter treatment with a moderately high level of commitment to giving it a try and who participate in and stay through the initial intensive inpatient or outpatient phases of rehabilitation. The best data on outcome for these men and women come from studies of alcoholics (1). Here, those people who entered care with some level of life stability (a family and job skills) and who fully participated and stayed through treatment have a two out of three chance (that's about 65%!) of staying clean and sober during the first year of follow-up. Few of the studies have carried the evaluation to five and ten years, but those that have done so indicate that the one-year rate of abstinence is likely to predict continued abstinence or at least extended periods without substances along with very short "slips."

The final bit of good news comes from the observation of the risk for severe medical or psychiatric conditions after abstinence is achieved (1, 2, 3). Several studies have shown that with continued abstinence, the levels of body and brain damage continued to improve every month. After extended periods of abstinence, the risk for high blood pressure, cancers, heart disease, and some forms of cognitive or thinking difficulties often approached the rates expected among non-substance-dependent people in the general population.

A Note to Family and Friends

What Can You Do During Treatment?

If you are reading this because you care about someone who is having some substance-related problems, I hope the information offered to this point will help you to understand what is likely to go on once that person begins rehabilitation. This and prior chapters have also been structured to give you the type of information that might be useful in helping the person you care about to choose between different types of programs in your community.

One aspect of this discussion that relates uniquely to you is the manner in which some programs work to incorporate relatives and friends into the rehabilitation phase of the treatment process. In general, the thinking is that substance dependence touches everyone within reach of the person involved. For example, the employer or teacher is affected by the types of behavioral changes almost certain to accompany repeated heavy substance intake by an employee or student. Similarly, friends who are not heavily involved with alcohol or drugs often cannot understand where the person's unpredictable behavior and explosive moods are coming from. Lastly, relatives suffer fears about lack of financial and emotional security in their lives; often, they have feelings of guilt regarding the possible role they might have played in the development of problems.

As a result, most treatment programs reach out to family members and friends. They offer education, problem-solving techniques, and counseling to those around the person with alcohol or drug problems. Similar to the approaches offered to the substance user, these steps include educational lectures, discussions, and films or videotapes appropriate for "significant others." If these are not given as an official part of the treatment package, family members and friends should ask about potential help. If not officially available, you can turn to self-help groups. Alcoholics Anonymous, for example, offers education and discussion groups for family members (Alanon) and for teenagers (Alateen). All you need to do is to pick up a phone book and call the AA number (no matter what drug problem is involved) and you can be referred to an appropriate group.

Sections of this chapter have discussed what goes on during sessions with the substance user, including the possibility of receiving family or couples counseling. I have also stressed the need to rebuild relationships while one is in recovery. Obviously, these issues relate to you as well.

What Is Codependency?

Sometimes, the treatment programs go a step further in dealing with family members. Many of these efforts fall under the jargon of dealing with **codependency**. As is true of much jargon, this means many different things to different people.

Being a partner or close friend or relative of somebody who is going through severe substance problems affects your life. This results in fears, frustrations, and subsequent arguments. Frequently, these fights include saying things that you later regret, which in turn generates more problems, and at times might help perpetuate the substance-taking behaviors.

Another related series of events often (not always) occurs in close relationships with people with substance problems. It doesn't take long for many people to realize that confronting the person with "using" and the associated behaviors (including lying, stealing, not coming home, and job-related difficulties) often results in an ugly scene. Sometimes, to avoid that pain, many people stop confronting the problems, and almost begin to accept the intoxicated behavior and its consequences as the normal course of life. This is quite understandable in human terms, but it does little to help stop the substance use problem.

Alternately, many people want to "rescue" those around them when troubles develop. Thus, when our children have problems at school, we want to help them with their homework or might blame the teacher or the school system for the bad grades. When someone we care about has a substance-related accident or suffers legal problems, our first reaction can be to jump in and try to lessen the damage. Although this is an understandable goal, unfortunately it can undercut someone's ability to generate enough anxiety and energy to stop using substances. After all, how can they convince themselves that they are in trouble and need to give up something important to them when every time trouble occurs somebody steps in the way and deflects the pain?

Codependency involves all of these issues, including arguments, behaviors that perpetuate use, and efforts to rescue. Self-help groups can help you to understand more about these problems and teach you how to deal with them in more effective ways. However, some health care providers do not work hard enough to be sure that family members realize they are not to blame for the substance use and should not feel guilty or responsible for the problems. Let me reassure you, therefore, that you are not uniquely to blame. Responsibility rests alone with the individual involved with substance-use problems.

There are many fine texts and self-help books available that deal with these complex issues. This chapter was written to help the substance user understand more about what is likely to go on as part of a rehabilitation effort. This is not a cookbook on how-to-do treatment but, rather, an overview of what to expect once treatment has begun. The same holds for the family.

A Recap

Rehabilitation sounds like a formal process. Actually, once you have recognized that a substance-related problem exists and have gathered up enough energy to try to do something about it, you have already accomplished 60% of what needs to be done.

The remainder involves letting other people help you to help yourself.

The process of recovery involves a series of commonsense steps aimed at helping you to achieve and maintain a high level of commitment to being clean and sober. If you know the dangers you face and have some understanding of the steps that can be taken to pull your way out of the quicksand, you will have the best chance of winning the battle to rebuild your life. This process of recovery involves education, discussions, observation of others who have gone through similar problems, and steps toward learning, relearning, and learning yet again.

Another essential step is to admit to yourself that staying clean and sober is far from easy. With sobriety you are giving up aspects of your life that are very important to you. Rebuilding a lifestyle without alcohol or drugs requires a careful commitment to a plan, learning how to use free time, reestablishing relationships, optimizing functioning at work and in social situations, and taking a host of other steps necessary to make you feel comfortable and at peace with yourself once again. This, too, is a process of learning and relearning over a period of many months.

This selection of the specific setting in which this process should occur is much less important than the actual process itself. The choices of inpatient versus outpatient care, rural versus urban programs, and medical or psychiatric or free-standing facilities are not the central issues. These details come naturally once you consider finances, the preferences of those around you, and the programs available in your community.

Of course, no one goes through life totally alone. Similarly, we do not face life problems or the need to rebuild in their wake without the consideration of family and friends. Therefore, it is not surprising that most treatment programs make concerted efforts to reach out to family and friends and to involve them in the recovery process.

Although the material offered in this chapter might sound simple, I never want to minimize the respect I hold for the dedication required by you and those around you to try to do something about a most difficult series of problems. I only hope that the information offered in this chapter helps you to recognize options that are available to you. After thinking about the material presented here, "rehabilitation" should no longer be a mystical word, but rather a fairly straightforward series of events that can take place in many different settings. No matter where it is carried out, successful treatment can only occur through your hard work and recognition that life can (and will) get better than it is now.

References

1. Sobell, L., Sobell, M., Toneatto, T., and Leo, G. What triggers the resolution of alcohol problems without treatment? *Alcohol: Clinical and Experimental Research* 17:217–224, 1993.
2. Klingemann, H. The motivation for change from problem alcohol and heroin use. *British Journal of Addiction* 86:727–744, 1991.
3. Bullock, K., Reed, R., and Grant, I. Reduced mortality risk in alcoholics who achieve long-term abstinence. *The Journal of the American Medical Association* 267:668–672, 1992.
4. Volpicelli, J., Alterman, A., Hayashida, M., and O'Brien, C. Naltrexone in the treatment of alcohol dependence. *Archives of General Psychiatry* 49:876 880, 1992.
5. Montgomery, H., Miller, W., and Tonigan, S. Differences among AA groups. *Journal of Studies on Alcohol* 54:502–504, 1993.
6. Ball, J., and Ross, A. *The Effectiveness of Methadone Maintenance Treatment.* New York, Springer-Verlag, 1991.
7. O'Malley, S. S., Jaffe, A., Chang, G., Schottenfeld, R. S., Myer, R. E., and Rounsaville, B. Naltrexone and coping skills therapy for alcohol dependence: A controlled study. *Archives of General Psychiatry* 49:881–887, 1992.
8. Meyer, R. E. New pharmacotherapies for cocaine dependence. *Archives of General Psychiatry* 49:900–904, 1992.

Additional Readings

Ancoli-Israel, S. *All I Want Is a Good Night's Sleep.* St. Louis: Mosby, 1996.

Bullock, K., Reed, R., and Grant, I. Reduced mortality risk in alcoholics who achieve long-term abstinence. *Journal of the American Medical Association* 267:668–672, 1992.

Fuller, R., Branchey, L., and Brightwell, D. Disulfiram treatment of alcoholism. *Journal of the American Medical Association* 256:1445–1449, 1986.

Klingemann, H. The motivation for change from problem alcohol and heroin use. *British Journal of Addiction* 86:727–744, 1991.

Montgomery, H., Miller, W., and Tonigan, S. Differences among AA groups: Implications for research. *Journal of Studies on Alcohol* 54:502–504, 1993.

Sobell, L., Sobell, M., Toneatto, T., and Leo, G. What triggers the resolution of alcohol problems without treatment? *Alcohol: Clinical and Experimental Research* 17:217–224, 1993.

Family Members and Friends

You might want to also turn to the references at the end of Chapter 6 and the general suggested readings at the end of Chapter 12.

10

What Happens Next?

Goals

By this point I have discussed all of the general lessons you need to know in order to rebuild a life free of substances. One of the rules that you have probably figured out for yourself is that there is a huge difference between learning about something and doing it.

This chapter discusses how to apply what you have learned. You already recognize that heavy doses of alcohol or drugs cause terrible problems in *anyone* and that for some reason you have a vulnerability to developing heavy substance use. Thus, in many ways you are special and run an extremely high risk of eventually developing severe problems whenever you allow yourself to use substances.

You probably found your way to this book because of a crisis that occurred in your life. If you have entered treatment, you were offered some combination of a good medical evaluation, detoxification if a physically addicting drug was involved, and counseling aimed at both keeping your motivation as high as possible and helping you to begin to rebuild your life without substances. These steps probably occurred through some combination of self-help groups, educational lectures, outreach to your family and friends, and individual and/or group counseling. Your personal "program" might have developed through any combination of meetings with a health-care professional, formal group sessions, and an inpatient or outpatient rehabilitation program. Therefore, an awful lot has been accomplished in the past weeks. Changing lifestyles, however, is not easy to accomplish. Starting to make changes is hard enough; keeping them going can be even tougher. This problem with maintaining change applies to people who diet to lose weight, those who have to alter their eating habits because of diabetes, men and women who must change their lifestyle following a heart attack, as well as for people attempting to minimize their risk of continued substance use problems. No matter which of these (or other) challenges are facing you, there are a number of questions you might be asking yourself. Some of these are reviewed in the following sections.

Why Do I Need to Continue to Get Help?

There are many clichés that apply here. The central issue, however, is that old behaviors are difficult to change. Therefore, we all require being taught, retaught, and educated yet again about how to accomplish long-term alterations in our lifestyles.

In the midst of the pain of a crisis, anyone is likely to be highly motivated to change the situation. People usually want to do everything possible to save their marriage, to avoid being thrown out of the house, to avoid losing a job or having to drop out of school, or to get out of trouble with the police. With the pain fresh in your mind, you are likely to be temporarily ultra-receptive to someone who tells you how to make the problem go away. As the pain fades as time passes, however, you might be less willing to pay the necessary price to keep things different from the way they used to be.

This "forgetting" the pain is probably a good thing in some settings. The ability to bury bad experiences is likely to help a woman decide to have a second child after a problem pregnancy and probably helps people facing multiple surgeries to go on to the next stage of care. However, for people with substance use problems, this self-protective mechanism backfires. Therefore, one important reason for requiring continued help over a period of time is the need to be reminded why it was so important to quit use of substances. Without the external help, you are likely to "forget" the pains, remember only the past pleasures, and lose your motivation for restructuring your lifestyle.

A related problem occurs when you look back and think that the recovery wasn't so tough after all. You are likely to be shocked at how "easy" withdrawal was and amused at how simple the lessons you have been taught appear to be. You tend to assume that because it was so "easy," maybe you don't really have a problem like "some of those other people." The next logical conclusion is that maybe you can take substances now and then.

Of course, if someone could only replay a videotape of the emotions and pain that accompanied the crisis caused by substances, and if it were possible to remember how many times you thought of beginning a "program" but backed out, you would be able to put some of these thoughts into perspective. But no videotapes of emotions are available. Therefore, you need continued contact with an aftercare program to keep the goals and reasons for abstinence fresh in your mind. Without aftercare, all the lessons learned are likely to be lost.

What's the "Best" Aftercare Program for Me?

You have already seen how there is no perfect and magical program for a person's recovery. So it should not be surprising that there is no single, essential way of carrying out aftercare. Once the more intense detoxification, rehabilitation, and the initial steps in a self-help program are achieved, the optimal continuation or aftercare program for you depends upon the same variety of factors that helped you to choose your program to begin with.

No matter what the final elements of this program are, almost everyone agrees that it is important not to depend only upon one approach. Because there is no "perfect" way to stay clean and sober, it is important that you use everything available to you to keep recovery going.

For most people, this means continuing in a self-help group such as AA. After the initial months of recovery, some men and women will use NA, CA, AA, or other groups almost daily, whereas others might continue on a once-a-week basis, increasing their participation at times when they feel more vulnerable to returning to substances such as when they are under stress or feel their craving increasing. Hopefully, most people *also* choose to continue in the aftercare program officially associated with their inpatient or outpatient rehabilitation.

This is not an either/or choice. It is probably best to combine the different approaches. There is also important help available from groups like Alanon that reach out to family members and friends, and similar groups are part of the aftercare component of almost all rehabilitation programs. Other people in recovery choose to incorporate formal aspects of religion, counseling aimed at helping with additional life problems, continued vocational rehabilitation, the use of exercise, and a variety of other procedures to help them feel more comfortable on a day-to-day basis.

So, what is the "best" program for you? I can give you a generalization: there are many potential components of an aftercare program, and it is up to you and your counselors to choose among them. However, I cannot offer a specific formula that states that X% of this and Y% of that must be applied to everybody.

How Long Does This Have to Go On?

As with everything that relates to recovery, this is a question that only you can answer. The most appropriate reply for you at this stage is that "it all depends."

Some of you will recognize the potentially disastrous results that are likely to occur if you go back to substance use. Therefore you are willing to devote a high amount of effort by attending aftercare meetings and working with a self-help group for as long a period as possible, as long as it decreases your chances of returning to substance-related problems. Others of you will decide that you enjoy the opportunity of "giving back some of what you got" by helping other people progress in their recovery. In either of those instances, you will probably participate in aftercare for somewhere between three and twelve months but actively maintain contact with your self-help group for a much more extended period of time. Your once- or twice-weekly (or even more frequent) Alcoholics Anonymous meeting, for example, will give you the chance to demonstrate to others who are just beginning to deal with substance-induced problems that recovery *can* be accomplished and that they are not alone. You might choose to become a sponsor where you are not only having an impact on the "group" but have one or more individuals you are trying to help on a more personal level. A sponsor is a specific person in the self-help group who becomes your advisor and teacher. He or she is the person you are likely to call when trouble looms or when you need advice.

Some of you, while extremely committed to recovery, find it important to put more of your efforts into your relationships with family members and friends. In this case, following the three to twelve months of aftercare and at least one year of active involvement with a self-help group, you might *decrease* (not stop) your interactions with AA, NA, or other related groups. Notice that I put an emphasis on the word decrease because most people working in the substance field believe that some sort of continued contact (even if only on a once a month or so basis) is an important way to continue to touch base with your peers and remind yourself that the minute you let your guard down regarding abstinence, there is a disaster waiting to happen.

Some of you are going to be tempted to withdraw from aftercare and AA or a related group as soon as you feel your life is coming back together. Although this decision will be up to you, retreating fully from an active recovery program is as unwise as stopping antibiotics too soon after pneumonia just because your fever decreased. If there really are formal stages of recovery, one of them almost certainly is a feeling of well-being that comes over people after they have passed that first obstacle and gone through the initial stages of active rehabilitation. This can be seen after one week or after six months or so; it all depends on the individual. We must remember that at this point, people are likely to have learned the lessons but to have had a limited opportunity to practice them. It is a very risky time to stop getting support. For almost everyone, a bare minimum of one year of continued contact with treatment and/or self-help groups is essential to maximizing the chance of continued recovery.

I know that life would be a lot easier if there were hard-and-fast rules about exactly what has to be done over precisely what period of time. Both the good and the bad news is that you have options—there are some decisions that have to be made. Each option has its own assets and liabilities. Whichever choice you make regarding the length of active participation in aftercare, however, I pray that you recognize the need to maintain contact on a regular basis with a mixture of self-help groups and an aftercare program for a minimum of twelve months from the time you leave your more intensive initial treatment.

How Can I Know if I Am Headed for Trouble Again?

Trouble is defined as anything that increases your risk for using again. Unfortunately, there are many dangers out there in the real world, and recovery requires keeping your guard up regarding your vulnerability toward substance use. There is a series of fairly common situations where your protective mechanisms have to be especially strong.

You Are in Trouble When You Think You've Really Got It Licked

When people begin to consider stopping substance use, they tend erroneously to picture a subsequent painful day-to-day fight where they are always under siege and never happy. This view probably reflects the many problems that have occurred in their lives related to substances. This awful and bleak picture also relates to how both drug and alcohol recovery are likely to be portrayed in the movies and on television.

Thank goodness that this is not the way things go! You will have moments when you are extremely proud of what you have been able to accomplish, times when you are overjoyed at how well life is going, and periods when your self-confidence is climbing. When these feelings occur, they are wonderful *as long as* they do not give you the idea that substance problems were not so terrible in the first place.

If you think about it and talk with people who were around when you were in trouble, there was a time when disasters were hitting you right and left. Although I would never recommend that you wallow in the pain of past problems, it is important to keep a level head that reminds you to be thankful that things are going well now, while at the same time never letting yourself forget how many problems you faced when you were using substances and how terrible things will become again if you go back to any substance use.

You Are in Trouble When You Find Yourself Interacting with Heavy-Drinking and Drug-Using Friends

It's not anyone's fault that you are likely to associate some person's face, voice, and demeanor with drugs and alcohol. On the other hand, these things happen, and you face great dangers of relapse to alcohol or drugs when you associate with people you identify with drug use and heavy drinking. Seeing and talking to these people will almost certainly increase your craving for alcohol or drugs. At the very least, interacting with heavy drinkers and drug users will increase the chances you have to start using again. The combination of the two factors, increased desire and increased availability of substances, does not bode well for continued recovery.

You Are in Trouble When You Allow the Day-to-Day Life Pressures to Build Up So That the "Old Feelings" Come Back Again

I have already told you that the usual alcohol- or drug-dependent person does not have a preexisting major psychiatric disorder. You are no more (nor any less) likely than anyone else to have had a major depression or anxiety disorder before substance problems escalated. However, once you got into heavy use of alcohol or drugs, the effects of these substances, along with the stressful lifestyle, were likely to have created lots of feelings of nervousness, frustration, and even hopelessness. Therefore, at least theoretically, these "bad feelings" might be closely intertwined in your mind with substance use.

The result is that when frustrations and tensions at home, work, or school get to the point that they are seriously bothering you, you might subconsciously connect these feelings with a need to use. Therefore, part of your recovery process should include exploring ways to handle these tensions and approaches that may give you a chance to deal with the problems before they reach crisis proportions. For our purposes here, when these frustrations are building, you are being given a sign that the danger of returning to drugs or alcohol is rising.

The three examples given above are only a few of the danger signs, but this list gives you the general picture.

What Do I Do if I Recognize the Dangers?

The jargon for what I am describing here is **relapse prevention,** a program briefly mentioned in Chapter 9 and formally discussed in much more detail by Drs. Alan Marlatt, Terry Gorski, and others (see the reference list at the end of this chapter). The goal of relapse prevention is to identify high-risk situations and then do something about them.

The philosophy requires steps that you need to take in order to know yourself and the situations around you well enough to be able to anticipate when you are at especially high risk for relapse. After acquiring the knowledge, you can then develop coping skills to decrease your chances of getting into trouble. The scheme is based on both learning appropriate thinking (or cognitive) strategies and practicing some straightforward behavioral techniques. Although the real beginning of a formal relapse-prevention program depends upon an interaction between you and a counselor, the basic idea makes great sense and can be briefly presented here.

Important aspects of continued recovery are learning how to anticipate and cope with feelings of craving for substances as well as dealing with urges to return to drinking and drug use. By paying attention to what is happening around you, perhaps even keeping a diary of feelings and events during the day, it is possible to identify situations where the urge to use substances increases. For many people, these high-risk situations involve feelings of anger and frustration, times of sadness or depression, situations in which anxiety increases, periods of sleeplessness, severe stresses at work or at home, encounters with specific neighborhoods or friends, and so on. Identifying high-risk situations not only allows you to avoid them whenever possible, but it also gives you a warning that it is time to put your guard up even higher than usual.

Before the craving or urge hits, it is possible to develop a plan to allow you to put the situation into perspective. One example is the need to see that the *urge for drugs comes on in a wave* that begins, rolls to a peak, and, with the passage of time, disappears. It is a time-limited occurrence and is not likely to remain active for hours and days—usually just moments.

Another component of relapse prevention is to recognize that the level of *motivation for abstinence is not always consistent,* and that, as with most important things in life, maintaining a high level of commitment to recovery requires active work. Therefore, when you find yourself feeling less committed to staying clean and sober, it is time to remind yourself about the situations that got you into the treatment process in the first place. This is a good time to think about the crises that occurred when you were using substances. It is also important to emphasize the gains you have achieved in your life since abstinence and to review which areas of your life are still precarious enough that a return to substances (with the accompanying destructive behavior) might result in a significant loss—a job, a spouse, and so on.

Relapse prevention also teaches you how some small and *apparently casual decisions* in your life are actually steps back on the road to using. Some of these choices include deciding you no longer need your AA sponsor, telling your spouse that his or her input is no longer needed in helping you cope on a day-to-day basis, finding yourself driving through the "old neighborhood," and agreeing to go to a party with a drinking or drug-using friend. In fact, every decision that increases the probability of the availability of substances, or puts you in contact with situations or people with whom you have used, can be part of a deliberate (although often less-than-conscious) decision to question your need for abstinence. Occasional but regular efforts to review where you are in your life and what decisions have recently been made are important steps toward keeping motivation and commitment to abstinence high.

So, there are a series of steps you can take to help yourself when dangers arise. Some of these are part of a formal approach to counseling called **relapse prevention.**

What Do I Do if I Slip (Find Myself Using)?

This is a very important question! The fact that someone would ask this demonstrates a good deal of sophistication about the process of recovery from substance problems. Here are some steps you can take.

Put the Slip into Proper Perspective

The answer to the overall question of how to handle slips is another important component of what you need to know to continue the maintenance phase of relapse prevention. The important first step here is to recognize that slips often occur during recovery but that they must be *placed into appropriate perspective*. Remember they are often temporary, usually occur during a specific situation, and are controllable. The psychologists who set up the relapse prevention approach point out the tendency many people have to assume falsely that the slip indicates something unique about them, something that is uncorrectable. Some people in recovery erroneously feel that a slip tells them they have lost the game. This thought process, formally labeled the **abstinence violation effect,** is often based on faulty reasoning.

In dealing with a slip it is important to remember:

1. A slip is not an inevitable sign of relapse and failure.
2. It does *not* wipe out all of the good things in your life that have developed during the period of abstinence. Those gains are real things you have accomplished.
3. While you *are* responsible for your actions, most slips occur in relationship to specific external events that can be changed.
4. There is no "domino effect" where the slip results in inevitable long-term substance use.
5. Most people around you have never noticed the slip—you are not the focus of everyone's attention.
6. The slip must be seen for what it is—an unfortunate occurrence, not a catastrophe.
7. Slips indicate nothing about your general level of willpower or ability to overcome a problem.

In fact, slips or lapses are *normal parts of the learning process*—they enable you to learn to keep motivation levels high and to establish a lifestyle free of substances. They are unique in time and in place. Indeed, a slip is undesirable, but it can be a valuable learning experience.

Once You Recognize You Have Used a Substance, Take Actions to Help Yourself

Once you have placed the slip into perspective, there are a number of steps that you can take. As soon a slip becomes apparent, *stop and reevaluate* where you are. Remind yourself to keep calm. It is appropriate at this time to review the reasons you chose abstinence in the first place. This will help you realize how important it is to stop substance use now. Look around you and try to *identify the specific situation* that seems to have contributed to the slip. Remember, both the present situation and the nature of substance use problems contributed to the slip. It is not that you have an uncontrollable problem.

At this point, *begin to use the detailed plan* for recovery you have developed as part of treatment. Steps you need to have worked out beforehand might include calling an AA or NA sponsor, attending a self-help group meeting, talking to your counselor or therapist, meditation, working on a hobby, taking on some additional task at work, and so on. In fact, it is not a bad idea for you to have written down your plan of attack to be used if a slip occurs and even to have rehearsed your approach through discussions with your counselor, sponsor, family members, or friends.

In this situation, there is an important game to recognize and to avoid. I don't know who started this, but somehow people seem to think that there is a magical clock of consecutive days of abstinence for which we are rewarded. The possible result of such thinking is that after a hundred days of abstinence, a slip means that all gains are lost and that you must start all over again. This can look like a monumental task because the person involved may feel that the "hundred days have gone to waste." *However, that is not how things work.* Your family and friends, your body, your brain, and psychological functioning all improve with the *total* number of days of abstinence you achieve, not just with consecutive days.

A slip means a *skip*, not a destruction of all that went before it. Several days of heavy drinking or drug use set everything back just that—several days. Even though a more intense effort at rehabilitation might be required for a time, you have still accomplished one hundred days of sobriety and being drug free, should be proud of that accomplishment, and need to recognize that so many of the lessons learned and the bridges rebuilt during that period of non-substance use still hold. You are one hundred days further along than you were before.

Therefore, a slip *is never an excuse for continued use.* You always have the option of going back to drugs and alcohol if you wish, but a slip is certainly not a license to do so. Slips are just a part of the recovery process for some people. For many of you, it is an indication that it is time to pick yourself up, dust yourself off, reevaluate the possible need for a more intense program for a period of time, and get on with the rest of your life.

A Note to Family and Friends

Things have come full circle. Earlier in this text I emphasized how, as family members and friends, you are not responsible for the alcohol or drug problem beginning in the first place. In a similar way, you were not the one who could make the decision to give up substances and enter recovery. Your job was to try to help the person to confront his or her own problems, to learn how to stop protecting the person from the consequences of substance use (or he or she would never quit), and make informed decisions about your own life.

After all that has happened, the rules have not changed. It is not your responsibility whether the person you care about actively works on a continuing recovery program. It is not your fault if your loved ones choose to go back to substance use. On the other hand, you can be honest and straightforward with them, helping them to recognize when problem situations have arisen and confronting them yet again if "slips" occur. If substance use resumes, it will be important for you to be on your guard to be certain that the substance user is never protected from the consequences of that use.

Many of you will choose to be very active in the continuing recovery process. You recognize how frustrating it can be when sobriety means that many of the old rules of interactions between you have changed. The fact that the person you care about is clean and sober now gives you the opportunity of trying to work through old emotions and complications while building a new relationship. The achievement of sobriety, however, does not automatically result in a smooth road. Much work still needs to be done.

Many of us need some guidance on how to reestablish communication, work through old resentments, develop trust, and strive to produce a comfortable and rewarding relationship. This help could come through formal counseling, might occur through interactions with a physician or clergyman, and might blossom through continued interactions with Alanon, Alateen, and other self-help groups. Personally, I would choose a combination of all of these approaches. The key here is our need for continued growth and additional advice as we are trying to work through where we have been, where we are, and where we want to be going.

Another important element should be considered. With the agreement of your family member or friend, it is a good idea for you to establish a specific staff person in the relevant treatment program with whom you will remain in contact. This individual can be of great help to you when and if you identify danger signs of a relapse as described above, or if a slip has occurred. It would also be a good idea to discuss with both your loved one or friend and a relevant advisor (in Alanon or from the treatment program) exactly what can be expected of you (and what you can expect of yourself) should problems develop.

A Recap

When you were a kid you might have played with a Mobius strip. This continuous curving ribbon of paper can represent how many important things in our lives have no obvious and clear-cut beginning and no formal end. In many ways, this is how I view substance-related problems. We live in a society full of stress and where alcohol and drugs are readily available. There is almost nothing any of you can do to isolate yourself totally from either stress or the availability of substances. Therefore, it makes sense that people who have had substance problems always carry a risk for recurrence of difficulties in the future.

No one deliberately made these problems happen. Some people in our society carry a higher vulnerability for heart disease, others seem to catch every flu that comes around, and yet others carry a higher risk for substance problems. The important steps are to recognize that the vulnerability is there, take care of substance-related problems when they occur, and recognize the need for active work in order to establish and maintain a recovery. Once the formal and intense "program" ends, you are in a position to be able to learn how to apply the important lessons to day-to-day life. This occurs through a series of trials (and I do mean trials) and challenges. The overall goal is to create the largest possible proportion of substance-free days for the rest of your life, with the hope that these will add up to 100% (or as close to it as possible).

In the same light, everyone's "program" is a bit different. Although active interaction with formal treatment or self-help groups for about a year is essential, and although some level of continued contact (perhaps on a less-intense basis) would be strongly advisable for the indefinite future, people develop different levels of interaction with these resources. Thus, some people, as well as their family members, will become very active and work to help others in the self-help groups. Others will choose to remind themselves of the need for extra work during periods of vulnerability using less frequent regular contacts with treatment and self-help programs.

The goal of this chapter was to remind you that, like the Mobius strip, recovery from any chronic problem is an unending process. I hope this text has given you some skills that have helped you enter recovery, begin to work things through, and recognize the need for continued effort.

Additional Readings

Birke, S., Edelmann, R., and Davis, P. An analysis of the abstinence violation effect in a sample of illicit drug users. *British Journal of Addiction* 85:1299–1307, 1990.

Daley, D., and Marlatt, G. Relapse prevention. In: Lowinson, J. H., Ruiz, P., Millman, R., and Langrod, J. (Eds.), *Substance Abuse: A Comprehensive Textbook*. Baltimore: Williams & Wilkins, 1992, pp. 533–542.

11

A Note to Family and Friends:
Pulling It All Together

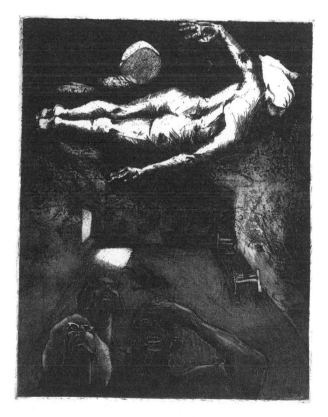

Figure 11.1. This illustration shows an individual soaring above the heads of three people on a clear moonlit evening. The thoughts communicated here relate to the interactions between the individual who is overcoming his or her life problems and those family members and friends who have lived through the process. In some ways, each person in this group is in the process of being released from a nightmare. The person going through recovery is in some ways by himself or herself but still functions as part of a unit. Chapter 11 brings together all of the lessons that this text has offered to family members and friends, those of you watching the process of transformation from a lifestyle dominated by alcohol and drug problems into a new set of much more hopeful life circumstances.

Goals

This book was written as much to meet **your** needs as to reflect the problems that might be faced by the person who has alcohol and drug problems. In order for you to be able to make decisions for yourself and to help the person involved, it is important that you have as much information as possible. So, Part I gave you a general overview of what drugs are and what they can do. You need this information to determine whether the pattern of use and problems are really worth concern. Then, Chapters 4 through 10 were written to help you see how you might actually help the person you care about get evaluation and treatment.

Sections at the end of Chapters 3 through 10 offered specific comments that emphasize issues from your perspective. A careful reading of each of these sections would give you all of the basic facts I think you need right now.

On the other hand, the information of use to you is spread throughout the text. If you are like me, at times of stress it can be difficult to focus your concentration and to fully understand things that are given in bits and pieces. Therefore, this chapter pulls together all of the individual bits of advice into a kind of review and overview.

The chapter is divided into two basic sections, with the first reviewing the major points chapter by chapter. The second section offers you some thoughts on a new topic that might be of some importance, namely a discussion of **how the information offered here impacts on young people in the family.** I hope some of that information might be of use in helping to prevent problems before they being.

An Overview of the Major Points Important to Family Members and Friends

Chapter by chapter, I have tried to increase an awareness of drug dangers, identify problem patterns that indicate a need for treatment, introduce the rehabilitation process, and describe what is required to stay clean and sober. These issues each impact on anyone who lives with or cares about someone with substance-related problems. These areas of concern for family members and friends of people with substance use disorders that are highlighted in Chapters 3 to 10 are briefly reviewed here.

Chapter 3

You can't make good decisions about whether you will invest more time and effort in staying with and trying to help someone with a drug or alcohol problem unless you understand what drugs are and the problems they can cause. Knowing whether a drug is physically addicting, understanding how the substance can produce mood swings or hallucinations, and recognizing the potentially deadly medical problems associated with substance use are also key tools you will need in order to confront the person you care about effectively. So, the material offered in Chapter 3 can be used by you when you attempt to establish a confrontation or intervention in which you can tell the person about your concerns. Chapter 3 also helps you to think about what life in the future might be like unless the person you care about stops all forms of alcohol and drug use.

Chapter 4

Even after understanding more about drug patterns and problems, many of us are tempted to believe that the people we care about are different somehow. They couldn't possibly be alcoholics or drug abusers because they are too nice, or too smart, or because they hold a job, or because we love them. A major road block standing in the way of our helping them is our misperception of what an alcoholic or drug-dependent person looks like.

Chapter 4 teaches you that most people who are dependent on substances do have jobs, families, and places to live. Men and women with substance-related difficulties are likely to attend our place of worship, be respected in the community, and be highly productive despite the severe substance-related problems. Their intake of alcohol and drugs is most likely to be an off-and-on again situation, with a period of control of use lasting days to months that almost inevitably leads to an increase in intake and a buildup of severe problems. The person with substance-related problems often recognizes that his life is not going well and develops successful (but temporary) efforts to stop or cut back substance use. This often produces an overriding pride in having accomplished the abstinence or new period of control. This pride leads to a conviction that if substance intake can be so "easily" altered, "there cannot really be a problem." Invariably, this "letting down of the guard" produces more substance use, and a pattern of severe difficulties soon develops. Thus, people who have repetitive alcohol and drug problems but who kept returning to use of the substance in the past have demonstrated a high likelihood (many would say an inevitability) of future problems if they go back to use. High levels of functioning and high moral standards do not make anyone immune to a substance-use disorder.

An important mechanism that contributes to the ability of a person with substance problems to keep going back to alcohol and drugs is the process of "denial." Here, it is likely that the person will blame everyone and everything other than alcohol and drugs for his life problems and will use these problems as an excuse for going back to substance use. In this regard, it is important for family members and friends to recognize how often this blaming type of behavior takes place and to avoid (as much as possible) having their own feelings hurt or convincing themselves that they, indeed, are a major cause of the substance problem. This is rarely the case.

Finally, it is important for you to work on avoiding your own case of "denial." Most people are tempted to look at the problems that develop in those around them and come up with excuses for their behaviors. You tend to believe that life would be better "if only" the person's job were more fulfilling, the person wasn't unemployed, she didn't have back pain, he hadn't been in Vietnam, and so on. You forget that other people with these same experiences and problems never develop severe alcohol- and drug-related problems. These life stresses and difficulties in themselves are not sufficient to cause a substance problem. Even if they contributed to the substance-related difficulties, the alcohol or drug intake is only likely to make matters worse. When intoxicated or hung over, it is very hard to work through and handle life problems. Nothing changes the fact that severe and repetitive life problems with substances predict future severe difficulties, no matter what the initial causes of the substance use disorder might have been.

In summary, family members and friends play a major role in trying to help the person with a substance use disorder to determine whether he or she has severe problems with alcohol and drugs. This requires helping the person to focus on the pattern of life problems, determining (to the best of one's abilities) if alcohol or drugs either caused or intensified the difficulties and to draw logical conclusions. Because we do not know the causes of alcoholism and drug abuse or dependence, all of the potential "excuses" of "I drink or use drugs because . . ." do not change the diagnosis. Present and past problems with substances predict future difficulties, no matter what other life stresses and challenges we have faced. Finally, it is important for everyone (you, me, and the person involved with substance problems) to recognize that anyone of any race, educational level, or socioeconomic group can develop severe enough problems from alcohol and drugs to need help.

Chapter 5

It is important to recognize that the causes of substance problems are very complex. It is almost certain that both environmental and genetic factors play a role. For a *small proportion* of men and women with substance problems, preexisting psychiatric disorders must be recognized and dealt with.

As discussed in both Chapters 5 and 6, sometimes, however, you assume that some factors caused the substance problems when they probably were not to blame. Substance use itself can cause physical problems (often as the result of accidents or damage by the alcohol or drugs to body organs) as well as terrible mood swings that, when caused by intoxication or withdrawal, can often be relieved by taking more of the substance. Heavy use of substances often causes you to pretty much put a "hold" on the continued development of personal relationships. Therefore, people with substance-related life difficulties are more likely than others to have chronic pain from injuries, to show failing health, to complain of many psychiatric symptoms including anxiety, depression, and even crazy thoughts or hallucinations, and to have problems with relationships.

Often, the person involved really believes that the alcohol or drug problems were caused by the pain or psychiatric symptoms. However, when careful research is done, about 80% of the time it is the other way around. Substances are likely to cause the life problems; there is little evidence that people with substance use disorders are more likely than others to have severe life problems before alcohol or drug problems began.

In any event, *even if* the medical or psychiatric problems came first, alcohol and drugs will only make the preexisting conditions worse. What is important here is to recognize that the first step in determining which came first is to stop all substance use and then reevaluate the symptoms. There is no way to deal appropriately with even real preexisting problems until full abstinence has been achieved and maintained for some weeks.

You can help your family member or friend to understand these issues. This type of information can be used by you in your confrontation of the substance problem, can help you to stop finding excuses for their substance-related behaviors, and can aid your efforts during treatment to help the person focus on the here-and-now as well as on a substance-free future.

One additional area of importance to you is raised both here and in Chapter 9. Because the person with substance-related life problems rarely lives in a vacuum, family members and friends are almost always asked to get involved in the treatment process. Usually, this involves several lectures or discussion groups structured for the family and friends, and these rarely include the person who is in treatment. Here, you will have the opportunity to learn more about the usual course and treatment for substance-related difficulties, and you can learn the steps you might take to increase the likelihood that treatment will be successful.

At the same time, any of you who have lived with people with substance problems remember situations in the past where you said things in arguments that you wish you could take back, avoided confrontations in part to "keep the peace," and even did things that might have helped to perpetuate the alcohol and drug problems. Sometimes, these steps that undercut sobriety were taken because you didn't "know better," and other situations might have occurred because you were angry. These are all human and understandable behaviors that happen in most people. In fact, these actions are so common that they are part of a larger (poorly defined) group of behaviors often called "codependency." A key step for family members and friends is to recognize the human nature involved in some of these actions. Once identified, it is possible to learn alternative ways of handling confrontations and day-to-day life stresses and to understand more about the recovery process.

In summary, family members and friends can play a very important role in the treatment of substance use problems. The information offered in Chapter 5 helps you to understand the difficulty in establishing "what caused what" in the course of substance problems. Sobriety can only make depression, anxiety, and pain syndromes better in the long run.

Chapter 6

Entering treatment can be very frightening. The more people understand about what is likely to happen during rehabilitation, the easier it is likely to begin care. You can be of great help here.

Chapter 6 teaches that there are only a few drugs that cause actual physical addiction, and even these produce withdrawal symptoms that are usually easy to treat. You can try to identify any specific fears that your family member or friend might have regarding how sick he or she might feel during drug withdrawal. You can be prepared to discuss that person's concern about problems sleeping, handling life stresses, and feeling humiliated if he or she goes into treatment. A key step in being able to stop substance use is learning to confront these fears, and you can help to identify questions that need to be asked of a care deliverer.

Making the intellectual decision to enter treatment often requires an additional bit of energy (sometimes supplied by family members and friends) to make that first phone call. So, it is worthwhile to review briefly where to get information and to have phone numbers and even specific names of counselors ready when the person you care about agrees it is time to learn more about how to stop substance use.

I also recognize that you are likely to have your own questions and need your own support group. That is why Chapter 6 tells you about the family and friend outreach programs of self-help groups such as AA as well as similar programs also offered by most treatment programs. These groups can be especially important in that frustrating situation where **you** recognize there is a problem **but your family member or friend does not.** These discussion groups can help you to make decisions for yourself and other family members, even if the person refuses to stop. The groups can also be a support when he or she enters care. Most groups remove a burden from your shoulders by reminding you that it is impossible to take responsibility for "rescuing" anyone. The groups can also give you more detailed advice about how to confront the person involved with substances. A brief script of what such an intervention might look like is offered within the "Family and Friends" section of that chapter.

Chapter 7

I can picture the frustration you must feel when you are in the middle of a crisis, have decided to get help for your family member or friend, but are unsure about how to select the "best" program. Because you are not likely to be a trained professional in the substance field, you might have the perception that there is an ideal treatment facility waiting out there and that if you choose the wrong one, the future is doomed.

Chapter 7 reminds you that treatment programs in the substance use area have more similarities than differences. In helping your family members or friends, you can remind them that the actual reason for choosing a specific program is often a matter of who happens to recommend what program to you, your finances, and the location of the program. Overall, I would recommend that you choose a treatment facility in the community where you live because of the ease with which aftercare can be arranged (see Chapter 10), and because selecting a local program maximizes the chance that family members and friends can participate in treatment. These practical considerations are usually more important than whether the treatment program is in a medical facility or stands on its own, independent of a major hospital, whether it is inpatient or outpatient, or whether the intensive phase of the program is for two, three, or four weeks.

Chapters 8 and 9

Too many family members see treatment as a magical black box. You know there is a terrible problem, you see the person walk in the door of the facility, you have brief visits during the intensive inpatient or outpatient phase of care, and see the person come out on the other side. Sometimes, not knowing what is happening on the "inside" creates fears that the staff is blaming family members and friends for the development of problems, or that staff would take upon themselves the responsibility of recommending the person to break off a relationship.

These two chapters offer both you and the individual involved with substances a chance to understand how treatment programs usually work. My goal is to describe the general plan in an effort to raise questions that you might want to have clarified, and to help you to recognize that no magic is involved—only hard work. I hope that understanding more about what the educational lectures are likely to cover and what issues are most often discussed in group and individual counseling will make it easier for you to talk about treatment progress with your family member or friend—and to ask staff members questions when they come to mind.

Chapter 9 also examines several areas where you can be of great help. It is important for you to recognize that one of the greatest challenges faced by a person recovering from substance problems is how to use free time appropriately and how to rebuild personal relationships. It is very frightening for the person in recovery to try to develop a new lifestyle when, in the past, so much of his or her time was engaged in getting substances, going through intoxication, and recovering from the effects of alcohol or drugs. To make matters even worse, it must be frightening for that person to force himself to sit down and talk with family members and friends when he is in the process of learning how much pain he caused those around him. For you as a relative or friend, understanding more about these issues through your own participation in self-help groups and groups sponsored by the treatment program is essential if you hope to develop some level of comfort, get rid of feelings of anxiety and anger, and begin to rebuild your own life.

Chapter 10

There is a simple message here. It is important for those around the individual with substance problems to realize that the intensive portion of outpatient care or the inpatient treatment approach can only begin to teach the lessons that need to be learned. Keeping motivation for abstinence high and rebuilding a life free of substances occur through a series of trials and errors. These can only be learned during real-life situations.

In effect, after the intensive phase of rehabilitation, the person with substance problems returns to the family, job or school, and friends, and he or she must learn how to cope with the associated stresses. This learning process requires continued support through ongoing contact with self-help groups and aftercare programs. This usually involves three to six months of relatively frequent involvement (often once to three times per week), after which each person has to consider the optimal level of continued contact. No matter what level is decided upon, some form of interaction with the treatment programs and self-help groups is important.

Chapter 10 also offers you some additional information. Although some people who are engaged in substance problems achieve abstinence and maintain it for the rest of their lives, most travel a rockier road. Slips do occur. Their possible appearance must be planned for and understood, and a scheme of steps to be taken if alcohol or drug use resumes should be developed. The approach is often called "relapse prevention," and the details offered within the chapter are important for you to keep in mind in helping your family member or friend to continue the process of rebuilding, even if a setback occurs.

Some General Thoughts on Prevention

Family members of people with substance use problems face a unique challenge. Although focused on helping the individual involved to recover and to stay clean and sober, as the initial crisis passes, they often turn their attention to other problems that might develop in the future. Because alcoholism is known to be genetically influenced, this raises the fear that other family members, especially the children, might be headed for trouble.

It is important to remember, however, that very little is known about the importance of genetic influences in abuse or dependence on substances other than alcohol. It is my guess that genetic factors do play a role, and that these might be almost as powerful as those involved with alcoholism, but it is impossible to be sure. I would also guess that if there are any genetic influences in developing dependence on heroin, cocaine, or other drugs, some of these factors might be different from those genetic influences that impact on alcoholism.

In any event, I can share some thoughts with you about prevention. These, basically, are some ways that I would approach potential problems in my children if alcoholism or other substance dependence problems had occurred within my family. These suggestions include:

1. Remember there is no predestination involved. People may enter life at higher risk for a substance problem, but the final development of difficulties is a combination of both genetics and environment.

2. Therefore, no one should ever throw up their hands and say: "It is written that I must develop these problems." In fact, people are born with all types of predispositions. Some are at high risk for diabetes, others for heart disease, and yet others carry a heightened risk for various forms of cancer. Each of us can take advantage of learning about our vulnerability by taking special precautions. For example, the individual with multiple relatives who have died of the same type of cancer should be especially careful about not smoking, avoiding exposure to environmental cancer-causing chemicals, and should have regular physical checkups. Thus, the person at risk for substance problems can recognize the risk and take appropriate steps to minimize the chance that alcoholism or drug abuse will develop.

3. I believe that children should be told about alcohol and drug problems that occurred in close relatives as soon as they are old enough to understand the concepts. You should consider telling your children that you or someone else close to them had a severe alcohol or drug problem. The more details you provide of the way in which these substances affected your life and the lives of other people the better.

4. An important part of this educational process is to remind the children that they are, of course, growing up in a society where alcohol and drugs are plentiful. Although these substances pose a danger to everyone, you should consider teaching your children that they may carry an especially high level of risk. As your sons and daughters grow older, it may be important for them to learn that children of alcoholics are four times more likely to develop severe substance problems themselves. It would be my guess that children of individuals with other severe substance use problems are similarly predisposed toward substance dependence. As discussed in Chapter 5, it might be appropriate to teach the children of alcoholics about the way that a decreased reaction to alcohol (an ability to drink other people "under the table") might not be something to be so proud of—it might actually herald a predisposition toward severe problems in the future.

Of course, no one knows how to prevent alcoholism and drug abuse. On the other hand, we can take advantage of the knowledge that alcoholism and drug dependencies run in families and that at least some severe substance disorders appear to be genetically influenced. Even if there are not enough data to be certain of the appropriate course to be taken within a family, it is my guess that the more the children know about the problems that have occurred in relatives, the greater their understanding of their own personal risk will be. The more they understand that they are responsible for their own actions (and that nothing is predestined), the greater the chance that they will escape substance-related problems.

A Recap

Many lessons taught in this text are as important for family members and friends of people with substance problems as they are for the people themselves. This chapter has pulled together information offered in Chapters 3 through 10 under the heading of "Family and Friends." I have tried to give you the opportunity to relearn some of the details that were expressed earlier within the text and to highlight specific sections that might be of special relevance to you.

Additional Readings

Bagnall, G. Alcohol education for 13 years olds—does it work? Results from a controlled evaluation. *British Journal of Addiction* 85:89–96, 1990.

Beresford, T., and Gomberg, E. *Alcohol and Aging*. New York: Oxford University Press, 1995.

Dryfoos, J. Preventing substance use: Rethinking strategies. *American Journal of Public Health* 83:793–795, 1993.

Ellickson, P., Bell, R., and McGuigan, K. Preventing adolescent drug use: Long-term results of a junior high program. *American Journal of Public Health* 83:856–861, 1993.

Ford, B. *Betty: An Awakening*. New York: Doubleday and Company, 1987.

Schuckit, M. Low level of response to alcohol as a predictor of future alcoholism. *American Journal of Psychiatry* 151:184–189, 1994.

Schuckit, M. A clinical model of genetic influences in alcohol dependence. *Journal of Studies on Alcohol* 55:5–17, 1994.

12

Some Concluding Thoughts

I wrote this book in response to situations in which people came to me for help, and I had nowhere to turn. The bookstores are loaded with fine and well-written texts that describe a specific treatment program, acquaint you with a self-help group such as Alcoholics Anonymous, or that share with you the stories of people who have faced problems similar to those described here and have learned to rebuild their lives.

The problem is that these books don't really accomplish what I need to have done. It is not always easy for people who have not been trained as professionals working in the alcohol and drug field to determine if a problem is present. Once a difficulty has been identified, if you don't know where to look, it can seem as if no help is available.

As is true of many books written for a general audience living in the real world beyond university and medical libraries, *Educating Yourself about Alcohol and Drugs: A People's Primer* was developed to help you make your way in the imperfect world in which we all must live. One of the pleasures that has come to me in writing this text is the fact that I now have a single reference to give to people who ask for more information about their own possible problems or as a consequence of their concern for someone significant to them.

It is important for you to remember that this is not a "do-it-yourself" manual. I don't believe that knowing more about whether a problem exists and understanding more about what happens in treatment give someone enough information to take care of their problem without help. At the same time, however, I hope that the thoughts offered in the prior eleven chapters will help you to make a rational decision regarding whether additional help might be required for a substance-related problem. These chapters were also written to make it a bit easier to think about getting help, by demystifying the process of treatment and recovery. Understanding more about what is likely to happen to you if and when you agree to get help can make that decision to seek treatment a bit less frightening. If even one person is helped through the information offered in this book, the effort was worthwhile.

This is a good time for me to try to make certain that I have expressed the major messages that the text has to offer in as clear a manner as possible. Most of the lessons I hope to have taught apply equally well to individuals who are concerned about their own possible alcohol- and drug-related problems and to those family members and loved ones who care about them. Some other messages deal more directly with the concerns likely to be expressed by family members and friends.

The most prominent general messages offered in this book include these:

1. All substances of abuse have their dangers. People experiment with alcohol and other drugs because of their desired effects, but (as is true with most things in life) there is a price that has to be paid.

2. The pattern of problems (or prices) related to the use of substances differs a bit between various categories of drugs. Therefore, it is important to place the substance with which you are concerned into a category or group based on whether it is a stimulant, depressant, opiate, marijuana-like drug, hallucinogen, inhalant, or any of a variety of other substances.

3. Everyone in life carries different types of vulnerabilities. Some people must limit their intake of lobster or other foods

because of allergies, others have to develop special diets because of their diabetes, and yet others are especially vulnerable toward cancers or heart disease. In each case there are subsequent important changes in their lifestyle that need to be taken to optimize their health. Those of you with substance use disorders also carry a level of vulnerability toward a life-threatening disease.

4. Although genetic factors play a role, no one fully understands why some people who use alcohol or experiment with other substances develop severe problems and others do not. The causes are likely to be multiple and complex. However, no matter what the original cause of the substance use problem might have been, the most important focus should be on how to develop abstinence and to maintain it while rebuilding your life without substances. The original causes (if they could ever be identified) have for years interacted with the levels of psychological and physical addiction to the drug and the lifestyles focusing on substance use—each of which tend to live on even if the initial cause was reversed.

5. Once you are involved in a substance use problem, the difficulties that you encounter affect many people around you. Therefore, it is important that your family members and friends know as much as possible about the usual course over time of substance use problems and the appropriate treatments. For this reason, the people who are important to you are often of great value to any treatment program in which you participate.

6. Only you can make the decision to stop substance use. Although your pattern of consumption of alcohol and drugs markedly effects other individuals, and even though the people around you can do a great deal to help you as you go through your recovery, it is your *own* commitment to recognizing the need to alter the direction in which your life is headed that is essential for recovery.

7. There are many ways to get help. All of the self-help groups, such as NA, CA, AA, and PA, are free. A number of organizations listed in the telephone book, including the National Council on Alcoholism, will give advice that is free. Those individ-

uals who are veterans and meet qualifications to be eligible for the delivery of care can receive free or at least reduced-cost treatments at Veterans Affairs Medical Centers. Almost all locales have city- or county-run outpatient or inpatient alcohol or drug detoxification or rehabilitation programs that are available at little or no cost. For those with insurance and with health care provided through government programs, there are a wide variety of potential treatments that can be sought out. Hopefully, this book has helped to outline where to begin.

8. There are many different options for treatment. Most outpatient and inpatient treatment programs offer a similar variety of mechanisms to help you. The choice of the facility in which you will receive care, the philosophy and training of the treatment personnel, and whether you will live at home or live in the facility during rehabilitation and detoxification rest with a variety of issues including cost, associated medical or psychiatric problems, as well as job and family pressures. It is important to recognize there is not a perfect program for you that must be sought out, but that you are likely to benefit from any of a variety of treatment approaches.

9. As you enter care, many of you will be surprised that the physical withdrawal symptoms are likely to be relatively mild, if they develop at all. You might also be amazed at how much common sense is used to dictate the steps that an individual needs to take in order to begin his or her process of recovery. Correcting the physical problems and learning the basic material are not usually what requires the most intensive work. It is the change in lifestyle, turning away from a focus on obtaining and using alcohol and other drugs to rebuilding neglected areas of your life with your families, hobbies, spiritual feelings, and your interactions with friends that dictate that recovery is a process that occurs over many months and often over many years.

10. Once you are fortunate enough to recognize that, more than anything else in the world, it is important to you to stop use of alcohol and drugs, you have taken a giant step forward. Your next giant step occurs when you recognize that you must

never let your guard down regarding your need to abstain. The original causes of the alcohol and drug problems have not been reversed, you have learned many reflexes that make you think of alcohol or drugs in a wide variety of situations, and for the rest of your life it is important to remember that substance use is dangerous for you.

Family members and friends can hopefully benefit from the ten points outlined above. In addition, there are a number of general themes specifically relevant to family members and friends that form the basis of much that is offered in Chapter 11 and in the sections at the end of most other chapters. These lessons include:

1. By learning everything that you can about alcohol and drug problems, you will be able to make the best possible decision regarding the way you might help the person you care about.

2. You did not cause the alcohol or drug problem in your friend or relative. Looking back, there may have been things you wish you had done differently, but this is part of the normal human condition and affects everyone. Still, it is important to remember that the complex causes involved in the development of alcohol- and drug-related difficulties are not likely to fall simply into the categories of the results of imperfect parenting, interpersonal problems, or the stress and concerns inherent in a parent–child relationship.

3. While considering offering help to the person with alcohol or drug problems, it is important that you make decisions regarding your own future. Therefore, the amount of support that you can offer your friend or family member is influenced in part by your own needs as well as the needs of other family members and friends.

4. Once you decide to offer help (either now or in the future) there are many resources available to you. It is essential that you remind yourself that you are not alone. There are many other people with alcohol- or drug-dependent relatives or friends, and these individuals need support and will benefit from interactions

with other people in similar circumstances. Therefore, Alanon, Alateen, and similar groups for relatives of drug-dependent individuals are all important resources for you.

5. Finally, recognize that recovery from alcohol- and drug-related problems is a *process*, not an event. The ability for the person with substance-related problems to recognize the difficulties or identify the role that substances have in these life problems often takes many confrontations, multiple consequences, and a great deal of time. Recovery begins with the recognition of the need for help, progresses through the treatment for detoxification (if needed), and only *begins* as part of the intensive inpatient or outpatient rehabilitation program. The real work of recovery requires returning to the day-to-day life situations and learning how to establish alternate ways of coping with stress and dealing with life's assets and liabilities while staying clear of alcohol and drugs. It is important for family members and friends to remember that it took many years for most substance use disorders to develop, and, similarly, it is likely to take a long period of hard work before an optimal substance-free lifestyle is accomplished.

I would like to conclude by reminding you that this book offers a variety of ways for you to learn more about the problems that are facing you or someone close to you. The most important advice is given through the words that make up the eleven chapters preceding this one. More information can be gathered through the references offered at the end of most of the chapters. These formed the basis for most of the conclusions and advice that make up the chapter material.

The final potential learning resource offered to you comes with the following list of *General Suggested Readings*. Here, I focus on general readings from other textbooks that might be of use if you feel you wish to study the general issues in greater depth. This general reading list is not as focused on specific material as is the case for the references offered at the end of most chapters. One of the *General Suggested Readings* is my own text. Since 1979, I have produced four editions of a handbook professionals can use for the identification, detoxification, and rehabilitation of individuals with alcohol and drug problems. This text has hundreds of references that document all of the major statements in great detail. The book is aimed at an audience of health care providers (from social workers through physicians), but it is listed here as a resource for you in case you need more detailed information. The remaining *General Suggested Readings* come from sources I often turn to in my own office.

General Suggested Readings

Edwards, G. *The Treatment of Drinking Problems: A Guide for the Helping Professions.* New York: McGraw-Hill, 1982.

Goodwin, D. *Is Alcoholism Hereditary,* Second Edition. New York: Ballantine Books, 1988.

Goodwin, D., and Guze, S. *Psychiatric Diagnosis,* Fifth Edition. New York: Oxford University Press, 1994.

Gossop, M. *Living with Drugs,* Third Edition. London: Wildwood House, 1993.

Ludwig, A. *Understanding The Alcoholic's Mind: The Nature of Craving and How to Control It.* New York: Oxford University Press, 1988.

Marlatt, G., and Gordon, J. *Relapse Prevention.* New York: Guilford Press, 1985.

Mendelson, J., and Mello, N. *Medical Diagnosis and Treatment of Alcoholism.* New York: McGraw-Hill, 1992.

National Institute on Alcohol Abuse and Alcoholism. Research Monograph 24, Alcohol and Interpersonal Violence: Fostering Multidisciplinary Perspectives. U.S. Department of Health and Human Services, 1992.

National Institute of Alcohol Abuse and Alcoholism. Research Monograph 25, Economics and the Prevention of Alcohol-Related Problems. U.S. Department of Health and Human Services, 1993.

National Institute on Drug Abuse. Research Monograph Series 72, Research Analysis and Utilization System: Relapse and Recovery in Drug Abuse. U.S. Department of Health and Human Services, 1986.

O'Brien, C., and Jaffe, J. *Addictive States: Association for Research in Nervous and Mental Disease*, Volume 70. New York: Raven Press, 1992.

Schuckit, M. *Drug and Alcohol Abuse: A Clinical Guide to Diagnosis and Treatment*, Fourth Edition. New York: Plenum Medical Book Company, 1995.

U.S. Department of Health and Human Services. Eighth Special Report to the U.S. Congress on Alcohol and Health, September 1993.

Vaillant, G. *The Natural History of Alcoholism: Causes, Patterns, and Paths to Recovery*. Cambridge: Harvard University Press, 1983.

Winger, G., Hofmann, F., and Woods, J. *A Handbook on Drugs and Alcohol Abuse: The Biomedical Aspects*. New York: Oxford University Press, 1992.

Wiseman, J. *The Other Half: Wives of Alcoholics and Their Social-Psychological Situation*. New York: Aldine De Gruyter, 1991.

References for Family and Friends

Johnson, V. *Intervention: How to Help Someone Who Doesn't Want Help*. Minneapolis: Johnson Institute Books, 1986.

Kaufman, E. *Help at Last: A Complete Guide to Coping with Chemically Dependent Men*. New York: Gardner Press, 1991.

A Brief Glossary

In writing this book, I have tried very hard to avoid technical jargon. All of the concepts involved in alcohol and drug dependence as well as in the rehabilitation of these conditions are relatively straightforward. Thus, there is no reason to hide behind scientific terminology.

Whenever a more technical phrase is used, it is defined within the text—at least the first time you see it. However, a short glossary with very brief (and thus not highly detailed) explanations of these terms might be of some use.

Abstinence Syndrome. This is also called withdrawal. After repeated intake of high doses of stimulants, depressants, or opiates, a subsequent decrease in the amount of the drug used can result in a syndrome that consists of symptoms that are usually the opposite of the original acute effects of the drug. For most substances, the more intense or acute abstinence syndrome is complete by about five to seven days; although a protracted abstinence syndrome of several months is likely to follow, it involves much more mild symptoms.

Addiction. This term is used to mean the same thing as dependence. It involves psychological and/or physical changes that occur with repeated intake of substances and contribute to a feeling of a need for the alcohol or drugs in order to feel comfortable. The various forms of dependence are described in more detail below.

AIDS. This abbreviation stands for acquired immunodeficiency syndrome, which comes from HIV virus infections and is often spread through contaminated blood present in needles or syringes shared by individuals using IV drugs.

Amotivational Syndrome. This feeling of a lack of ability to focus or concentrate and lack of motivation to carry out day-to-day tasks (at work and/or school) is probably a consequence of the active ingredients of marijuana remaining in the body for many days after intoxication.

Bacterial Endocarditis. This consequence of the IV injection of material contaminated with some types of bacteria involves an infection of the internal lining and the valves of the heart. This can result in heart failure and death and is one potential consequence of IV drug use involving nonsterile needles and syringes.

Benzodiazepines. These are a type of brain depressants that cause a high and have a pattern of problems similar to alcohol. Within the text, these are also referred to as the Valium-like drugs.

Blackout. This is a condition of forgetting all or part of what had occurred during a period of intoxication when the individual was awake and alert. This is seen primarily with the brain depressants including the benzodiazepines and alcohol.

Codependence. This is not an actual syndrome; the term codependence is used to describe characteristic ways of adjusting and interacting with the family member or friend who has a substance use disorder.

Convulsion. The text refers only to full or grand mal convulsions where an individual rapidly loses consciousness, at first becomes very stiff with rigid muscles, and then, after a minute or so, develops rhythmic jerking of the arms and legs. This can be observed during an overdose from various drugs like cocaine or amphetamines and is sometimes (but rarely) seen during withdrawal syndromes from alcohol or other depressant drugs.

Denial. As used in this text, this is a process of either not recognizing or refusing to admit the relationship between substance use and severe associated life problems.

Dependence. This term is used to mean the same as addiction as described above. The term dependence is used three ways in this text. First, it is used to indicate psychological feelings of discomfort when the drug is not available (psychological dependence). Second, it can indicate the abstinence or withdrawal syndrome that is likely to develop when depressants, stimulants, and opiates are rapidly stopped. And third, dependence can indicate a definition of a more severe substance-related problem—for example, alcohol dependence, which is generally used to mean the same thing as alcoholism.

Flashback. This is an unwanted recurrence of a drug high that is experienced hours or even days after the drug was taken and the individual had recovered from intoxication. This condition, which will disappear on its own with time, has been reported to occur with the marijuana-type drugs and the hallucinogens.

HIV. This abbreviation stands for the human immunodeficiency virus that causes AIDS.

Hepatitis. This literally means an inflammation of the liver. The toxic effects of alcohol on the liver can cause an alcoholic hepatitis, while a virus spread in contaminated blood through shared needles among IV users causes an infectious type of hepatitis.

IV. This means intravenous use or the administration of a drug through a needle directly into a vein.

Neurotransmitters. These are chemicals in the brain and in other parts of the nervous system that are released by one nerve cell to subsequently attach to structures (receptors) on a nearby nerve cell in order to stimulate that second cell. The neurotransmitters mentioned in this text include the chemicals dopamine, serotonin, norepinephrine, and GABA.

Peripheral Neuropathy. This syndrome involves a destruction of the nerves to the hands and feet with associated numbness and tingling as well as "pins-and-needles" sensations. It can be caused by a variety of conditions but is often a consequence of very heavy long-term alcohol use.

Physical Addiction. This concept is described above under addiction and dependence.

Psychological Addiction. This is described above under addiction or dependence.

Receptors. As used here, these are structures that exist on the outside of nerve cells and that respond to the stimulation caused by neurotransmitters. The result is stimulation of the cell to which the receptor is attached.

Snorting. As used here, this means taking a drug by inhaling it into the nose. This is also called insufflation.

About the Author

Marc Alan Schuckit, M.D., is a professor of psychiatry at the University of California, San Diego School of Medicine and is director of the Alcohol Research Center, San Diego Veterans Affairs Medical Center. He also serves as the director of both the alcohol and drug treatment program of the San Diego Veterans Hospital and of the Scripps McDonald program affiliated with the Scripps Memorial Hospital. Dr. Schuckit has an active research career and is the author of over 350 scientific publications, including the textbook *Drug and Alcohol Abuse: A Clinical Guide to Diagnosis and Treatment* (Plenum), now in its fourth edition. He is the editor of the *Journal of Studies on Alcohol* and has served on the editorial boards of the majority of internationally significant alcohol and drug journals.

Dr. Schuckit has received many awards and honors, including the American Psychiatric Association's Hofheimer Prize for research, the Distinguished Scientist Award of the Research Society on Alcoholism, the Mark Keller Honorary Lecture Award from the National Institute of Alcohol and Alcohol Disease, and the Isaacson Award from the International Society of Biomedical Research on Alcoholism. He is a fellow of the American Psychiatric Association, American College of Neuropsychopharmacology, and the West Coast College of Biological Psychiatry.

Index